Sleep
and your
Special
Needs
Child

In the same series

The Journey Through Assessment:
Help for Parents with a Special Needs Child

Food and Your Special Needs Child

Sleep
and your
Special
Needs
Child

Antonia Chitty
Victoria Dawson

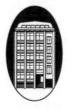

ROBERT HALE • LONDON

© Antonia Chitty and Victoria Dawson 2014
First published in Great Britain 2014

ISBN 978-0-7198-0791-6

Robert Hale Limited
Clerkenwell House
Clerkenwell Green
London EC1R 0HT

www.halebooks.com

All content within this book is provided for general information only, and
should not be treated as a substitute for the medical advice of your own doctor
or another healthcare professional. Case study names have been changed.

A catalogue record for this book is available from the British Library

2 4 6 8 10 9 7 5 3 1

Typeset by e-type, Liverpool
Printed in Great Britain by Berforts Information Press Ltd

Contents

Introduction

Sleep issues for children with special needs are extremely common. If you are reading this book, the chances are that broken sleep has become a chronic issue for you, your child and possibly the whole family. Only once you have experienced long-term sleep interruptions can you truly understand the effects it can have on your health and well-being.

As a new parent you may have expected a few months of broken nights before your baby began to settle, but as a parent of a child with special needs you may be struggling with sleep issues that seem never-ending. Almost nine out of ten children with additional needs have sleep problems, so if you care for a child with sleep difficulties you are not alone.

Don't feel that you are failing if your child has sleep issues. Many children with additional needs take longer to learn to go to sleep and need more help with their sleeping routine than others. There may also be medical, social and sensory issues that impact on the quality of your child's sleep.

In this book, you can learn about the different type of sleep issues and find out more about specific conditions and disabilities and how they affect sleep. You will discover advice from experts and case studies where parents share their experiences and what has worked for them. Read on to find out about good sleep practices too, and positive ways to encourage your child to sleep through the night. Discover plans for bedtime routines, and learn about when medication might help.

Sleep is vital for our children's well-being. Without enough sleep their health, mood, behaviour and learning ability will all be affected. Research suggests that children with additional needs are more likely to have sleep disorders and, for these children, sleep problems are persistent, and are not likely to improve without intervention.

Statistics suggest that 41% of children aged four to twelve years in special schools have difficulties settling at bedtime, compared to 27% of children in mainstream schools. Children with additional needs also seem to have greater difficulty staying asleep (45% compared with 13% of children in mainstream school). Children with severe learning disabilities are even more susceptible to sleep difficulties with over 80% of children up to the age of eleven years demonstrating sleep problems. Research also suggests that children who have autism are more likely to have sleep difficulties and this is reported to be between 34% and 80% of children with a diagnosis.

This is a pressing issue for parents: disturbed sleep causes depression, relationship problems and even weakening of the immune system, impacting on both mental and physical health. While parents of babies expect sleep problems to resolve within months, parents of children with special needs can find these problems lasting into adolescence and beyond. Research has shown that addressing these problems using a behavioural and cognitive approach to sleep management is highly successful, because many sleep problems have a behavioural basis. A different approach is needed if your child's sleep issues have, for example, a medical basis, so getting to the root of the problem is vital.

The majority of parents receive little or no help around sleep problems other than medication. Few families have access to sleep practitioners in the United Kingdom unless they can afford to see one privately. The practical advice in this book will help parents to feel more in control and more confident about tackling sleep issues in a way that is appropriate to their child.

Resolving behaviour-based sleep problems can be challenging and it is important to identify what the difficulties may be so that you can choose appropriate strategies: this book will show you how.

Chapter 1
The Importance of Sleep

How sleep helps your child

Sleep is vital for every child. Good sleep can help physical development, and a solid night's sleep contributes to every child's mental and
emotional well-being. According to The Children's Sleep Charity:

" *Children and babies who get the right amount of sleep are
more likely to:*

- *Be mentally alert*
- *Have a brain that functions better*
- *Have sharpened senses*
- *Be able to learn to their full potential*
- *Be happy and pleasant in disposition*
- *Concentrate*
- *Do better in school*

Sleep helps our bodies to develop by:

- *Supporting our immune systems*
- *Releasing hormones that aid growth*
- *Helping tissues to repair*
- *Leaving us feeling better* "

What happens when you get disturbed sleep

Sleep deprivation has more effect than you might imagine. When you
always get a good night's sleep you have little understanding of what
lack of sleep, night after night, can do.

The effects of sleep deprivation on your child

Children who don't get enough sleep can fail to reach their full potential in many ways. Lack of sleep can make it more difficult for a child to deal with emotional challenges, leading to behavioural problems. Lack of sleep damages concentration, which can affect a child's ability to learn. Some children lack energy when they don't get enough sleep, but others become hyperactive. It is easy to get into a cycle of daytime naps and broken night-time sleep. Lack of sleep can even impact on a child's appetite and growth.

How siblings can be affected

Lack of sleep for just one family member can affect all the family. On the simplest level, night-time noises can wake your child's siblings, particularly if they need to share a bedroom. Sleep-deprived children can be more fractious and clash with siblings too. Siblings can end up with similar issues to those listed in the paragraph above, even though their disturbed sleep is secondary. Sleep disturbance can also impact on family activities: you may decide against letting the sibling have a friend to sleep over, for example. The Children's Sleep Charity says, 'Siblings comes up as a massive issue in our workshops. Visit www.sibs.org.uk for support for siblings of children with special needs.'

✓ Sleep deprivation affects the whole family:
✓ Relationship breakdowns: marriage/family/siblings/parent-child
✓ Arguments
✓ Resentment (between all!)
✓ A rollercoaster of emotions: hatred, anger, blame, depression, teary
✓ Loss of earnings
✓ Accidents
✓ Illness
✓ Isolation
✓ Inability to cope with other roles/demands in life
✓ Stressful
✓ Inability to think rationally

(reproduced with permission of The Children's Sleep Charity)

Sleep deprivation as a parent

As a parent, sleep deprivation can be exhausting. Your child may have a range of needs that you have to deal with: dealing with these day in, day out, on insufficient sleep can push any parent over the edge.

If your sleep is disturbed, you can find this affects your memory and concentration too. You can struggle to know whether you are making good decisions and feel emotional or angry. Loss of sleep can lead to issues with anxiety and depression, and, in the long term, you can find yourself falling ill more often too.

What's more, every parent needs a little child-free time when the children are asleep. If you can't count on your little one to nap, or find every evening is a series of trips up and down stairs to settle your child, you miss out on important time to recharge your batteries and relax.

You may find that your relationship suffers too. Heightened emotions and too little quality time together will affect even the strongest relationships and parents of children with additional needs can find their relationships in difficulty for these reasons. You may never get to sleep with your partner if you take turns to look after your child at night, or one of you ends up staying with the child.

The sleep cycle and the different stages of sleep

Do you understand what happens when we sleep? We think of sleep as a singular activity, but in fact it is made up of different phases. Understanding these phases can help you work out what is causing your child's sleep issues.

Sleep helps your child grow and stay healthy. During sleep, growth hormones are released, the immune system works hard, and the brain processes data from the day. This backs up our memory and concentration powers. During sleep the body repairs itself both physically and mentally.

Sleep has different stages, made up of REM (rapid eye movement) and non-REM sleep. Non-REM sleep breaks down into stages 1, 2 and 3. Stage 1 sleep is the lightest sleep, when you are just dropping off. Stage 2 is deeper than stage 1. Stage 3 is the deepest sleep, during which you may struggle to wake. During the early part of the night your child may experience stages 1, 2 and 3, but as the night goes on they may just cycle through stages 1 and 2. Night terrors and sleep-walking can occur when coming out of stage 3 sleep.

REM sleep happens around ninety minutes after we fall asleep, and is the phase where we dream. You may see your child's eyes moving rapidly under their eyelids when they are experiencing REM sleep. The brain is active but the body cannot move.

From three months of age, each sleep cycle lasts about ninety minutes. Your child is most likely to awaken between cycles. It takes about ten minutes for children and older babies to fall into a deep sleep. Toddlers and babies spend a lot of time in this sort of sleep. During this period, the body switches off and the brain receives extra blood and processes the day's events. Non-REM sleep only develops when a baby is four months old. This is the time when sleep becomes restful and muscles relax. The body is repaired by non-REM sleep. We experience this series of sleep stages several times each night. When we move between stages we experience what is known as partial waking. Often we are not aware of these partial wakings; we simply turn over and go back to sleep.

A complete sleep cycle is when we pass through the three stages of non-REM sleep and the stage of REM sleep; sleep cycles vary in length depending on the age of your child. They may last less than an hour in infants while young people will have a sleep cycle lasting around nintey minutes. See the table on page 18 for more information regarding how long your child may need to sleep each night.

Partial waking

Everyone wakes partially in the night, but we usually go back to sleep without realizing this. Children who have not learned to settle themselves, however, may wake fully at this point. There are things that may make it more likely that a child will wake. The Children's Sleep Charity says:

> " *A child who partially wakes in a different environment to the one where they fell asleep may fully awake. For example, if your child fell asleep on the sofa downstairs and you carried them upstairs to bed, they may experience a partial waking*

and then go on to wake up fully as their environment has changed. Just imagine if you fell asleep in bed and then partially awoke and found yourself in another room, you would wake up startled too! 〕〕

Our body clocks

Our body temperature and hormones change throughout the day; our bodies have what is referred to as a circadian rhythm. It is this that indicates to our bodies when it is time to be awake and when it is time to go to sleep. This cycle runs over a period of twenty-four hours and takes its cue from daylight and darkness.

Research has found that if we are deprived of light our circadian rhythm runs at a little over twenty-four hours. This is important to note if your child has a severe visual impairment and is not able to respond to light; sometimes these children are prescribed melatonin to help to support their body clock.

Melatonin

Melatonin is a hormone that occurs naturally in our bodies. It is produced at night and helps us to go to sleep. Darkness helps to promote the production of melatonin; this is why it is a good idea to put your child to sleep in a darkened room. There is some research that suggests that kids with ASD don't release enough melatonin and that in children with ADHD release is delayed.

Melatonin is sometimes prescribed to help with sleep difficulties. Even if your child is prescribed melatonin you should still maintain a good bedtime routine and follow the advice in this book around sleep hygiene. Melatonin will only work if all other conditions for sleep are correct, e.g. your child is tired, comfortable, in a quiet, dark room, not hungry or over-tired and feeling relaxed. It may help your child to go to sleep but doesn't help keep them asleep.

Case study

Carly's son, Tim, was born with a left-sided congenital diaphragmatic hernia (CDH) which was corrected by surgery at Great Ormond

Street Hospital when he was eighteen days old. He has had kidney problems, digestive problems and breathing problems. Tim is now ten, and Carly says, 'We still deal with glue ear, a poor immune system and occasional fainting/scary stopping-breathing incidents. He also has a speech and language impairment, dyspraxia, sensory regulation disorder, memory problems and auditory processing disorder. Tim has a combination of issues with his sleep.' Carly explains: 'As a consequence of CDH he has chronic abdominal pain, and occasional sickness at night when food can't pass a "kink" in his bowel while he is lying down. He also wakes with night sweats: he soaks the bedding and we have to change it. And sometimes he will appear to wake, and be disorientated but unable to communicate."

Tim's difficult start meant that in his first year he only slept for two hours at a time. Carly says:

" *By the time he was ten months I was a wreck! I turned in my car keys to my husband, explaining I was seeing things and felt I shouldn't drive. In hindsight I think this was caused by the terrible start to Tim's life. Hospital procedures require regular observations; I completely understand the reasons for this but I remember holding in a scream of frustration when I had just managed to get him to sleep and another nurse walked in to poke and prod him. He was an incredibly light sleeper; any noise or movement used to wake him – if he fell asleep in the car he would instantly wake the minute the car stopped or the engine turned off. This leads on to the second problem – he would not sleep well during the day unless he was in his cot at home. The early two-hour sleeping pattern we addressed with ghastly control crying at about ten months old. It was really hard emotionally but we took it steady, followed the method in Toddler Taming, using lots of going back in to reassure but setting out firm boundaries – and again gritted our teeth. I have used this with all my kids at some point or other. Both the girls were sorted in about five days, Tim took fourteen days but at the end of it we were all better off! Tim then slept fiveish hours at a time at night so was only waking once or twice a night – it was a vast improvement all round.* "

Tim has always been an early riser. Carly says, '5 a.m. starts were the real low point! Most days he now wakes up around 6.30 a.m. but we have taught him to play quietly in his room for a while. He also falls into/out of sleep patterns very easily. Two late nights close together will cause us trouble with settling him the following night.' Carly finds her daughters are much less disrupted. The lack of sleep affects Tim, and his education. Carly explains, 'On bad days, Tim is grumpy, less willing to do anything, and less able to cope with sensory input, which is already an issue for him. Therefore, we see a marked increase in the number and duration of meltdowns when he is tired. His school report states that he is less focused, more tearful, complains of headaches and is more likely to refuse social interaction.'

Carly has noticed something that makes Tim's sleep worse:

   A stressful bedtime – I know it sounds obvious but we really notice it; if we are absolutely calm and in control, he relaxes; if I'm upset or get cross, things go wrong on a sliding scale. Watching films/programmes in bed is also not good – we have tried it in desperation! Tim may fall asleep during it but will usually wake before midnight and, even if he doesn't, he is more tired the next day. I think this is a hard one for parents – it's the immediately easier path when they ask for a film before or during bedtime – they get ready for bed really fast and with less resistance – but I think it very quickly becomes a problem because there is no way I would read to Tim for as long as the duration of a film. In our case the worst thing we can do is make Tim go to bed on a full stomach – we're just asking for it then! Ironically I find it's worse if he's over-tired already.

Tim's specific problem with vomiting in the night happens if he eats shortly before going to bed. Carly explains how they have worked on this:

   We carefully manage meal times. Tim can't go to most after-school events because he must have his dinner before 6 p.m. If I'm to work till 5 p.m. then collect him there isn't time to cook a good dinner. Therefore we use the majority of Tim's DLA money to pay for an after-school nanny to collect all three kids from school. She is able to sort out any immediate issues with the school, has been trained to help Tim with his evening OT and schoolwork and also gets dinner on the table for 5 p.m. She is worth her weight in gold! 〞

Carly has been affected by Tim's sleeping patterns. She says:

〝 *Lack of sleep makes me clumsy, irritable and unable to see options and alternatives. I gave up my job and now work for myself. I put on weight, made mistakes at work or when out and about. I rarely go out or see friends, my husband cannot stay awake during a film! I find I get more illnesses and bugs hit you harder. Part of my difficulty is that even when Tim does sleep there is so much to organize around his care and schooling I often lose sleep reading reports, writing emails to the school or therapists or just through the sheer stress of issues up in the air. There aren't enough hours in the day to manage the whole caboodle of parenting, job, housework, other stuff that crops up like car issues, house maintenance and then the management that comes with a multi-therapy child plus all their therapy! Inevitably it eats into precious sleep hours.* 〞

Tim's sleep issues have got better as he has grown up, even if they are not totally resolved. Carly says:

〝 *I used to start to feel stressed from about 5 p.m. onwards. I learnt not to try and delay it – bad, bad move! Since our nanny started in September 2011, life has improved hugely. She gets the ball rolling three days a week by sorting dinner on time so when I walk in from work I'm oddly fresh for the run-up to bed and keen to see the kids and hear about their day. In the past, the day-in, day-out drudgery of the same post-4 p.m. arguments used to mean I was wrung out by 7 p.m. and desperate for the cavalry (husband) to arrive to help with bedtime. I used to dread that first bit of getting them up the stairs for a bath.* 〞

Carly has some tips for parents in a similar situation:

✓ Aim for a good, regular, calm bedtime. It is hard to do but really does help.
✓ Find out whether your child has any real risks to health that prevent you from sorting their sleeping out.
✓ Think about the space they are going to sleep in – start thinking about what you need to relax and go to sleep (when you're not exhausted, that is) and then layer over the top any issues you know your child has. Then create that space (and the time every day for your child to use it).
✓ Catch up on sleep when you can… if you can get some relief during the day, take it!
✓ On a bad day, seek comforting support: call a friend round for coffee, call your mum, forgive yourself the housework and muddle through, but start aiming for a better bedtime this night from as early as possible.

How much sleep does your child need?

Different children need very different amounts of sleep, but there are guidelines that will help you decide whether your child is getting approximately what they need.

Up to one year

Your baby's sleep requirements change drastically during their first year. Initially they will sleep for around sixteen hours in every twenty-four, with a regular cycle of sleeping for an hour or two and then feeding. Soon, though, as the baby's stomach grows and their needs develop, they can sleep for slightly longer periods, and have longer periods of being awake. By the end of their first year a baby will be sleeping for around eleven-and-a-half hours at night, with around two-and-a-half hours' nap time during the day.

ISIS (the Infant Sleep Information Source) provides information about babies' sleep based on a variety of research. The website provides factsheets about infants sleep, and you can read in-depth information by logging on to www.isisonline.org.uk.

Toddlers and pre-schoolers

Toddlers need to nap too: different children will drop their naps at different stages, but most will drop their need for a nap by the time they are four. Daytime naps will tend to shorten in duration, so while a child may need to sleep for more than two hours at twelve months, by three years they should be napping for just an hour.

At the same time as naps shorten, toddlers will continue to sleep for a little over eleven hours per night. During this phase there are still many reasons that a child will wake in the night and need a parent's reassurance to settle again. Dropping naps will increase the amount of time your child sleeps at night: a pre-school child of four who doesn't nap may need eleven-and-a-half hours of sleep per night. Don't be tempted to cut your child's naps too soon, though. See below for more about naps.

School-age children

As children grow from five to ten years their need for sleep diminishes slowly and gradually. While your 5-year-old may need eleven hours of sleep, a ten-year-old may only need nine-and-three-quarter hours. By fourteen years this could be down to nine hours as the need for sleep reduces around fifteen minutes for each year of age. Remember that each child's needs varies, and can depend on their level of activity, but the general trend should be true for all.

How much sleep?

Every person is an individual. Therefore the following table should simply be used as a guide to how much sleep may be needed:

Age	Average daytime nap	Average night-time sleep
3 months	5 hours	10 hours
12 months	2.5 hours	11.5 hours
3 years	1 hour	11 hours
6 years	None	10.5 hours
9 years	None	10 hours

This table is reprinted with permission from The Children's Sleep Charity

Moving into adulthood, your child will need between seven-and-a-half and nine hours sleep each night.

Daytime naps

Young children need to nap during the day so they don't become over-tired. According to The Children's Sleep Charity, naps can help children sleep better at night. The charity advises:

" *Try to get your child to nap in their cot or bed. Do not try to stop your baby napping in the daytime; a sleep-deprived baby will be over-tired and may take longer to settle at night. Log your child's naps in a sleep diary so that you can work out how long they are napping each day. Space your child's naps out so that they get the full benefit from them. The daytime sleep cycle is forty-five minutes so to get the full benefit of a nap your child should be encouraged to sleep for at least one sleep cycle.* "

Lack of naps can make your child appear hyperactive. Encourage your child to nap until they reach two to three years.

Nap tips from The Children's Sleep Charity:

" • *Make sure that you have set nap times so that your child gets into a routine*
• *Wind down with relaxing activities prior to nap time such as a cuddle and a story*
• *Make sure that your child is comfortable, fed, changed and that the room is at the correct temperature*
• *Let them settle themselves to sleep, even if they do not nod off they will benefit from the rest* "

Children with special needs may continue to nap even past the age of two to three, but for some older children, naps can become a problem. According to The Children's Sleep Charity:

" *Sometimes older children may take naps during the day that they don't really need. This can mean that they do not sleep well at night because they simply are not tired. Keeping a sleep diary is helpful for noting the number of naps that a child has. If your child is at school or accesses school transport it is useful to ask the staff whether your child is napping during the day. This helps to build up an accurate profile of the amount of sleep that your child is getting.* **）】**

Why children with additional needs may have sleep problems

Children with additional needs are more likely to have sleep issues than other children. Your child may experience physical discomfort which keeps them awake. Some medications can cause disturbed sleep. Sensory issues can cause sleep problems: a child with sight loss and no perception of light, for example, may struggle with the difference between day and night.

Many children with learning difficulties can take longer than you would expect to learn to self-settle. This doesn't simply affect the child at bedtime. As you have read with regard to sleep cycles, we go through phases of deeper and lighter sleep during the night. Children may wake during the phases of light sleep and be unable to get themselves back to sleep again. Behavioural issues may also impact on a child's ability and desire to go back to sleep.

Finally, if your child has breaks in routine for hospitalization this can lead to disturbed sleep.

Sarah's sons both have conditions that cause broken sleep. She says:

（（ *Richard has now finally been diagnosed with chronic ADHD. His medication has affected his sleep. It makes going to bed no problem but he is waking up at 3 a.m. regular as clockwork! He finds it hard to get back to sleep until around 4 a.m. Michael has Asperger's; he is fifteen, not medicated. He is currently having night terrors and when returning to sleep the dream picks up where it left off... As a result he won't go back to sleep! He tends to be awake about 5 a.m.* **）】**

We'll look at this in more depth in Chapter 2.

Keeping a sleep diary

Keeping a sleep diary is an important first step to improving your child's sleep. You can use the diary to note down what your child has been doing during the day, and how they sleep afterwards. This allows you to see whether different activities help or hinder a good night's sleep.

Here is an example:

Child's name: Jamie			Date: Jan 23		Age: 3		
	DAY 1	DAY 2	DAY 3	DAY 4	DAY 5	DAY 6	DAY 7
What you did during the day/afternoon	Nursery	Park, followed by playgroup	Nursery	Nursery	Day at home, went to supermarket	Play date with friends	Doctor's appointment first thing, then at home
Any naps during the day? Write down the time of nap and how long your child slept	20 mins – 9 a.m. 2 hours – 3 p.m.	1 hour – 9 a.m. 2 hours – 4 p.m.	2 hours – 7 a.m. 1.5 hours – 3 p.m.	20 mins – 9 a.m. 2 hours – 3 p.m.	2 hours – 7 a.m. 2 hours – 4 p.m.	1 hour – 10 a.m. 2 hours – 4.30 p.m.	2 hours – 4 p.m.
What your child ate/drank for the evening meal	Sausages and beans at 5.15 p.m. with milk	Shepherd's pie 6.15 p.m. with milk	Beans on toast 5.50 p.m. with milk	Spaghetti Bolognese at 5.15 p.m. with milk	Refused dinner, then had a snack with us when we ate dinner at 8 p.m.	Refused dinner, then had a snack with us at 8 p.m.	Refused dinner, then had a snack with us at 8 p.m.
Any medication taken?	None	None	None	None	None	None	None
Time bedtime routine started?	7 p.m.	8.30 p.m.	7.30 p.m.	8 p.m.	9 p.m.	9.45 p.m.	10 p.m.
Time your child was in bed?	10 p.m.	11 p.m.	10.30 p.m.	9 p.m.	10 p.m.	10 p.m.	10.30 p.m.
Did you stay or did they self-settle? Write your comments here	I stayed	I stayed	I stayed	I put TV on but had to go back	I stayed	I put TV on but had to go back	I stayed

	DAY 1	DAY 2	DAY 3	DAY 4	DAY 5	DAY 6	DAY 7
Time your child went to sleep?	11 p.m.	Midnight	11.30 p.m.	10 p.m.	10.30 p.m.	10.45 p.m.	11 p.m.
When your child woke during the night, how long were they awake/where did they go back to sleep? (Your bed/their bed etc.)	Woke at 1.30 a.m. Up for an hour. Went back to sleep in my bed	Woke at 2.30 a.m. Came in my bed and went to sleep after half an hour	Woke at 2 a.m. Came in my bed and slept straight away	Woke at 12.30 a.m. Came in my bed and slept after an hour	Woke at midnight. Came in my bed and slept straight away	Woke at 1 a.m., sat with him for an hour until he slept.	Woke at 12.30 a.m., came in my bed and slept immediately. Woke again at 3.30 a.m. for an hour
When your child woke in the morning	7 a.m.	7.30 a.m.	7 a.m.	6 a.m.	7 a.m.	6.30 a.m.	7.30 a.m.
Total hours slept (including daytime naps)	9.5 hours	10.5 hours	11 hours	10.5 hours	11.5 hours	10 hours	10.5 hours

Now, are you ready to keep your own sleep diary? It will help you work out why your child is missing out on a solid night's sleep. Here are some tips to help:

✓ Keep the diary by your bed – this way you are more likely to fill it in at the time and get the details accurate

✓ It doesn't matter what day you start the diary on, simply fill in day 1 and move through the week. Print out two sheets to create a diary for 2 weeks

✓ If the diary isn't large enough simply make additional notes on a separate sheet

✓ Please be honest when filling in the diary

✓ If you can't face filling it in during the night then invest in a Dictaphone and record the night waking. The next day you can simply transfer the information onto the diary

✓ If your child stays elsewhere make sure that you send the diary so that you can see if they sleep differently in different environments

✓ Share the diary with practitioners and see if they can identify any patterns

Summing up

Having read this chapter, it is now time to review what you have learnt about children and sleep.

It probably isn't news to you that disturbed sleep can cause problems for the whole family. On the other hand, a good night's sleep can make everything seem easier. Work through the recommendations in this book and see how to help your child.

Remember that older children need to learn to settle themselves to sleep. For children with additional needs this may take longer than you expect. Sleep has different phases, and it is common for children to wake fully in the lighter phases. Helping your child to learn to self-settle is important. Read on for more about helping your child to settle in Chapter 2.

Your child's need for sleep will change as they grow. Young children need to nap during the day, and it is important not to cut naps too soon. Many children will continue to nap even past the age of two or three. If your child doesn't sleep at night, yet naps a lot during the day, shortening their naps may be one strategy; see if it helps. Start keeping a sleep diary to see whether this could be an issue for your child.

Children with special needs may have a complex range of issues that affect their ability to go to sleep and remain asleep. Physical pain can cause night waking. If your child has health issues, the issues themselves or the medication your child needs to help with the issue can cause sleep problems. See Chapters 3 and 4 for more on medication and sleep. Behavioural issues can cause problems with going to sleep and also leave your child lacking the resources to go back to sleep during the night. Again, a sleep diary can help you identify where problems might be arising.

Finally, if you are trying to improve your child's sleep and coping with broken nights at the same time, remember that everything will seem doubly hard. Hang in there; things will improve as you work your way through the advice in the next chapters.

Overleaf is a blank sleep diary for you to use.

Child's Name:	Date:		Child's DOB:

	DAY 1	DAY 2	DAY 3
What you did during the day/afternoon			
Any naps during the day? Write down the time of nap and how long your child slept			
What your child ate/drank for the evening meal			
Any medication taken?			
Time bedtime routine started?			
Time your child was in bed?			
How your child settled – time taken to fall asleep etc. Did you stay or did they self-settle?			
Time your child went to sleep			
When your child woke during the night, how long were they awake/where did they go back to sleep? (Your bed/their bed etc.)			
When your child woke in the morning			
Total hours slept			

DAY 4	DAY 5	DAY 6	DAY 7

Chapter 2
Sleep Difficulties

Introduction

This chapter is where we start looking in more depth into the range of issues that can stop children sleeping. Sleep problems are more common in disabled children and those with special needs, and these children also have more difficulty staying asleep. This is especially true of children with severe learning disabilities: over 80% of children in this group up to the age of eleven years demonstrate sleep problems.[1]

Different conditions have links to sleep issues. Research has found that between 34% and 80% of children diagnosed with ASD have sleep problems.[2] Another study compared children with typical development to those with ASD and those with Asperger's disorder. The children with Asperger's showed more symptoms of sleep disturbance, and different types of sleep problems than those with ASD, and both had more sleep problems than those with typical development.[3] You can read more about how specific conditions link to sleep issues in Chapter 9.

For children with additional needs, sleep problems last seven years or more, and usually need some sort of intervention to resolve.[4]

If you have completed the sleep diary in Chapter 1, you may have more of an idea of what is causing your child's sleep issues. If you have not yet completed a sleep diary, go back to Chapter 1 and copy out the diary or find a notebook and start making notes about your child's sleep. This will help you identify causes of sleep issues, and learn from the points in this chapter. Unless you find out 'why' your child has problems sleeping you can't find the right strategies to deal with it. Sometimes there may be a number of possible reasons why, so you need to identify the reasons and then work from there. Read on to find out more about possible causes for sleep issues.

Sleep disturbances can be caused by physical problems – for example, a child may be unable to get comfortable due to a physical impairment or medical condition. Behavioural issues are the leading cause of sleep problems, as the way a child behaves can seriously hinder their ability to fall asleep or stay asleep. Some children with conditions that lead to delayed development may continue feeding during the night: this can also be the case for children with digestive disorders who may need supplementary night feeding.

Many children with sleep issues also have anxiety problems: this can become a cycle where the brain is too active to sleep, the child gets used to struggling to go to sleep, and then becomes anxious about not sleeping. Anxiety problems are particularly common for children on the autism spectrum, but can affect any child.

Some sleep problems occur when the child does not develop a routine of winding down before bed, settling themselves to sleep and resettling as they enter lighter phases of sleep. They can end up taking most of the evening to fall asleep, going to the parents' bed when they wake, or simply continuing to wake frequently well past baby- and toddlerhood.

All of these issues, along with very early waking, can cause lack of sleep for parents, with detrimental effects on your relationships, health and well-being. Add in parental anxiety around your child's medical issues and you can end up with sleep problems of your own.

That is a very quick round up of some of the issues covered in this chapter. For each issue, you will find some simple strategies to try yourself to improve things, and suggestions of what to do when you need further help.

Physical issues

There are a number of reasons why your child may not be sleeping. If you can identify what is causing your child's problem you can then work on strategies to try to improve the situation. Reasons for your child not sleeping could include the following. Read the tips along-side each, and use the suggested strategies to help:

✓ *Is your child too hot or too cold?* This can wake children in the night. If you go to your child and they have woken, how do they feel? A young child who kicks their covers off may prefer a sleeping bag: an older child may be better off with several layers of sheets and blankets rather than a duvet. You may also want to adjust the heating temperature and the time it goes off and on. Finally, a fan may help during hot weather: make sure it is out of your child's reach though.

✓ *Is your child hungry or thirsty?* If your child wakes because they have digested all their food and are ready for breakfast, or feel thirsty in the night, a little planning ahead can help. Make sure that your child is eating enough before bed. Chapter 4 has more advice about food and sleep.

✓ *Is your child wet or soiled?* If your child is disturbed by the need to wee or a wet nappy, try cutting back on drinks in the hour or two before bed. Make sure they use the loo before bed too. You may want to purchase nappies designed for night-time use, which may stay dry for longer. And if your child is able, explain that they can get up, use the loo, and go back to sleep. Leave a night light on to light the way to the bathroom if you need to.

✓ *Is your child unwell or in pain?* If your child's medical condition or disability causes problems during the night, speak to your GP or specialist. There are a number of medications that can help children sleep better, and an adjustment to the way your child's medication is given may also help: for example, slow release tablets can sustain their effect. Read more about this at the end of Chapter 4. Many children can cope with pain when distracted during the day, but find it is more of a problem at night. If your child is woken by discomfort, you need to consider their pain relief: again, talk to the specialist or pharmacist. Teething is a specific cause of pain.

✓ *Is your child being woken by light?* Try blackout blinds. You can improvise with card, a thick towel or a blanket. EasyBlinds (www.easyblindsonline.co.uk) has a wide range of permanent and temporary blinds for all sizes and shapes of window. Read more about blinds and the bedroom setting in Chapter 6.

✓ *Is your child being woken by noise?* You may have a delivery truck that rumbles past every morning, a noisy milkman, or other noises that disturb your child. Consider whether a white noise machine would block out some sounds, or even see whether another room in the house is quieter. Again, there is more about this in Chapter 6.

You may also want to consider whether your child is over-stimulated by their bedroom environment: read Chapter 6 for more about this topic.

Behavioural issues

Many, many sleep issues can be described as 'behavioural'. This includes children who don't want to get into bed, those who don't want to stay in bed, those who struggle to settle themselves to sleep, those who wake in the night and those who rise early.

Child behaviour expert Jane Cross of Behaviour Advice says:

" *I find that sleep-related issues are nearly always down to lack of routine and inconsistency. Even when parents or carers think they have a regular routine, on closer analysis there are inconsistencies that can be smoothed out. Even children with ADHD-type behaviours can be coaxed to relax and stay in their rooms. My experience is that old-fashioned advice such as sticking to a routine, with time to unwind, a bath, stories, calming music and soft light and sticking to this routine nearly always works.* "

In the following section we will look at different behaviours, what's behind them, and how you can address them.

Children who don't want to get into bed

Do you have a child who hates going to bed? One who fights to stay downstairs when you tell them it is time to go up?

Amanda is mum to Rory, aged fourteen. Rory was born fifteen weeks prematurely and suffered lung and brain haemorrhaging as a result. This left him with cerebral palsy and hydrocephalus. He is right-sided hemiplegic and is most likely autistic: he is going through the assessment process at the moment. Because of Rory's autistic tendencies he has ended up with a specific bedtime routine. Amanda explains:

" *When it's time for him to go to bed, he likes to watch a DVD or play on his iPad in bed to help him settle. However, he likes to have things a certain way. He used to insist that I took him to bed so we would have to go through this act every night where he would send my husband into the kitchen for his drink and we would 'sneak' upstairs to bed, leaving my husband to shout, 'Where did they go?' This came about after we did it once only and it took a long time to wean him off it. We did that on his eleventh birthday when we convinced him that he was a big boy now and could take himself to bed.*

Now he does go upstairs and gets his pyjamas on by himself but he still likes to have a snack – a bagel, perhaps, or a toasted muffin – with a glass of cordial. He will shout down shortly after he goes to bed for the snack and then he will come down with his plate if he eats it. After that, he will come down if his iPad is out of charge, or if he has run out of juice, even if he isn't going to drink it. Often we have found a full glass still there in the morning because he has asked for it just before falling asleep. He leans the iPad on the wall and watches a movie on it while he falls asleep. It takes him longer to settle if something isn't making some kind of noise. He likes to have a light on. Once he is asleep he tends to stay asleep though. "

Amanda adds:

" *He will settle perfectly fine if he has what he needs, but if any-thing is missing he will take longer. If he is sent to bed with a snack and juice and iPad he is fine. I think the whole muffin/juice thing is just a way of getting us to go to him (he can't carry it upstairs by himself). Maybe I'm too soft with him but I figure he has enough problems so if he wants me to take him a snack and a drink then I will.* "

This difficulty in settling has an impact on Rory at school. Amanda says:

66 *He attends mainstream school for two days a week and special school for three days. It is difficult to get him up for school if he has taken a long time to settle the night before. There have even been occasions when the school has asked us to pick him up because 'he's not quite himself today' and once in the last year he has fallen asleep in class. He can get tired easily and will fall asleep in the car on the way home if he has been to bed late the night before and he has had a particularly tiring day. It has been like this for a few years.* 99

Louisa says:

66 *Adrian always used to fight bedtime, so we came up with several strategies to help. It has been an ongoing issue for us as he is totally immune to reward systems. Before he could read we used to start a story CD for him. Now we offer unlimited reading time with an endless supply of new books. We have a strict rule that unless there is blood or vomit we don't want to see him again until morning, and to that end, he has a note pad in his room to write down anything vitally important that he previously felt he must, must tell me there and then!* 99

HOW TO HELP
Start a regular pre-bedtime routine. Sarah says:

66 *We have a helpful tip for getting the children to go to bed. Around five minutes before bedtime David gets a yellow card which shows him he has a few minutes left, then the red card shows him it is time to stop what he is doing, choose the toy he wants to sleep with, and go up to bed.* 99

This card system is also in use at David's school, so he is used to it for all sorts of activities.

A routine will help your child get prepared for bed mentally as well as physically. Start the routine at the same time each night: this will have roll-on benefits as they will wake at the same time in the morning too. Be firm: this is a time of the day when you need to stick to your guns. If your child needs assistance in understanding when their time is up you could use a card system like Sarah, or buy a sand timer so that they have a visible reminder that their playtime is coming to an end.

EXAMPLE OF A BEDTIME ROUTINE

Start with thirty to sixty minutes of quiet time before bed. This is time for books and jigsaws. Switch off computers, the TV and other electronics. Quiet music may help some children with a sound cue that it is wind-down time.

Next, it is time for a bath or shower. Look at child-friendly bath products with lavender in to help your child relax. Nell, who is mum to three, says, 'James always appreciates bath time: he gets some time away from his siblings and calms down.'

After bath, it is time for pyjamas, tooth-brushing, and one last trip to the toilet. Reading a story to your child at bedtime can also have many benefits. It gives them a positive reason to get into bed, plus important quiet time with just you. Then, kiss your child goodnight and leave the bedroom. At this point many children try to stall for time – one more kiss, one more drink, etc.: as a parent you are probably familiar with this sort of request. Be prepared. If your child always asks for a drink make sure they have their water bottle by the bed. Be firm but gentle and don't give in! Read more about bedtime routines in Chapter 5.

WHAT TIME SHOULD YOU SWITCH OFF THE LIGHT?

In order to work out when your child should go to bed, go back to Chapter 1 and see how much sleep your child might need at their particular age. What time do you want them to wake up? Allow for daytime naps if your child still needs them, and this should help you work out the right time for your child to go to sleep. Do remember that if your child has a condition that means they expend less energy, such as impaired mobility, they may need less sleep too.

Examples:

If your 6-year-old child needs ten-and-a-half hours of sleep and you want them to wake at 7 a.m., their lights should go off at 8.30 p.m.

If your 3-year-old needs twelve hours of sleep and has a one hour nap, they should go to sleep at 8 p.m. to wake at 7 a.m.

Remember that children's sleep needs can vary depending on activity: for example, 4- and 5-year-olds may suddenly start going to sleep earlier once they have started school.

Some children have developed delayed sleep phases where they don't nod off until midnight and then they sleep until mid-morning. If this is the case you need to strengthen your child's body clock by putting them to bed at the time they are genuinely tired. So put them to bed at midnight and begin the bedtime routine at 11 p.m. Move the routine and bedtime forwards by fifteen minutes every couple of nights. Gradually their circadian rhythm will strengthen so that they are tired at an earlier time.

TOP BEDTIME ROUTINE TIPS FOR PARENTS AND CARERS

✓ If your bedtime routine is not working, call in reinforcements. If your child is 'much better for Grandma', for example, ask Grandma to put him or her to bed and watch and see what happens

✓ If you struggle at bedtime because you have been with the children all day, ask your partner to take a turn

✓ If you are hungry, tired and cross after a long and difficult day, give yourself five minutes off, and have a cup of tea and a biscuit before starting the routine: if you are relaxed, everything will go better

✓ If you are struggling at the moment with exhaustion, just make one small change that you feel comfortable with. You can gradually implement change over a period of time. It is better to make one small change and stick with it than to make a whole load of changes and then not have the capacity to carry them through

Sula says:

> **❝** *We offer stickers for good going to bed and a reward for gaining so many stickers. I give him a set of conditions that he has to meet. The three conditions are the time he has to go to bed, the time he has to switch off his TV and that he has to go to sleep without any fuss. If he meets all three he gains a sticker. Then when he has reached a month's worth of stickers he gains £5. We stick the stickers on a chart, and I have the conditions he has to meet written on it. Also you can get music specially for children's bedtime. It is piano music that you play in the background and it promotes relaxation. John Levine has a whole range of music. I've used it with myself and recommended it to others. I have seen a great improvement at bedtime with these ideas.* **❞**

Children who don't want to stay in bed

Do you have a child who won't stay in bed? This section is about the child who yo-yos up and down stairs till 11 p.m. Later in this chapter we'll look at the one who sneaks into your bed at 3 a.m.

Some children just drop off to sleep. A story, a kiss, and two minutes later they are soundly asleep. If you are reading this book, the chances are that this doesn't happen for your child. The child who pops out of bed is generally one who finds it hard to go to sleep. This could be for a range of reasons: physical discomfort has been addressed already in this chapter, so now we will look at behavioural issues. And don't forget to look at how much sleep your child is getting: just not needing to sleep at the time they go to bed can be an issue. Most children take fifteen to twenty minutes to fall asleep, so for some children it is a question of ensuring that they are sufficiently relaxed, warm and comfortable in their bed to ensure that they want to stay there.

Some children find it hard to switch off and relax. Follow the tips on page 33 to improve your bedtime routine. Switch off stimulating activities at least an hour before bed. This might mean the computer, handheld computer games, the TV, or homework that needs to be done well before bed. Also, make sure there is time during the day for your child to share their thoughts and worries, as some children tend to save them all up for bedtime!

Try teaching your child simple relaxation techniques to help them settle into sleep more easily. You can get books and CDs that will help you, incorporating a relaxing bedtime story and simple breathing exercises. See the Relax Kids range, for example, at www.relaxkids.com or on Amazon.

Some children struggle to stay in bed because their bedroom is just too full of interesting stuff to do! If your child likes to get up and play, add 'packing away the toys' to the bedtime routine. If your child has a TV or computer in their bedroom, can you move it elsewhere? See Chapter 6 for more tips on creating a relaxing bedroom environment.

Other children may be too interested in what is going on elsewhere in the house. It can be hard if your child has older siblings, but try to keep the noise down for half an hour after bedtime: have the TV on low or use headphones. A child who is used to fighting sleep will tend to look for distractions, and if they can hear what you are up to they may come and investigate.

Nell says:

" *My boys share a bedroom, but there are four years between them, so James was keeping Kris up. They have very different sleep needs too. Kris goes to sleep earlier and wakes up earlier than James. Things have worked better at bedtime since I started putting James in the bath while Kris is dropping off to sleep rather than trying to get them both into bed at the same time when James didn't need to go to sleep that early.* "

Children who struggle to settle themselves to sleep

Many children with additional needs and/or disabilities can have had difficult starts in life. Going to sleep on your own, or 'self-settling', is a learned skill: your child may have had disruption, such as a hospital stay, at a time when they might otherwise have been learning this skill or they may have delayed development that means that they have not yet learnt it. There are a number of strategies to help you teach your child to self-settle.

Start with your calming bedtime routine, as above. Kiss your child goodnight, switch the lights off and leave the room. This will give them a chance to fall asleep on their own. If your child does not currently go to sleep without you, and if they are able to understand, explain what will happen under this new system.

For some children, you may decide on a more gradual approach, e.g.:

- ✓ If you usually hold your child while they drop off, sit beside them
- ✓ If you usually sit on the bed, sit on a chair. Each evening you try this you can move the chair a little further from the bed
- ✓ If you always sleep with your child, you could try putting a mattress next to your child's bed instead. Again, you can gradually increase the gap between you

Stay clear of your child's bedroom for fifteen to twenty minutes to avoid making noises which could distract and wake them. If your child gets up, put them back to bed calmly, and tell them to go to sleep. Ideally, each time you will be spending longer out of the room. Be calm, quiet and boring if you need to talk to your child. This may take a number of nights, but it will improve your child's ability to self-settle. If you and your child continue to struggle it may be time to get professional help. See the resources section for ideas and contact details for professionals.

Children who wake in the night

Everyone has phases of deep and lighter sleep: see Chapter 1 for a fuller explanation of the phases of sleep. Babies and young children may wake fully during the lighter phases of sleep while adults and older children will stay asleep. The age at which your child 'sleeps though' without waking will vary from child to child, and additional needs, physical illnesses or disabilities can affect this further.

When you understand that everyone enters lighter phases of sleep, you will be able to see that the child who struggles to self-settle is likely to wake and be unable to get themselves back to sleep, while the child who is used to dropping off to sleep by themselves may rouse but fall asleep again easily. If your child knows you were alongside them when they dropped off, they may be alarmed if you are not there when they wake, whether it is ten at night, one in the morning or breakfast time. Children may cry out at this point, whether to call for you or simply because they are expressing distress at being alone and are unable to go back to sleep; children who can walk unaided may get up to find you at this stage.

Nell says:

" *James always used to get up in the night, around two, and come and climb into our bed. I was a bit worried that this would carry on: when he was two and a half I became pregnant and didn't really want to be feeding the baby in the night as well as having a toddler in bed. I was happy with co-sleeping up to a point, but struggled with lack of sleep myself with wriggly little ones in bed with me. James could just drop off back to sleep, while I lay awake. My husband used to end up sleeping on the sofa too, which wasn't great. In fact, James woke less and less, and was sleeping through by the time the baby arrived. James is now seven and his little brother nearly four, and Kris is doing the same thing. I try reminding him to stay in his own bed before he goes to sleep at night, but in the middle of the night I'm too tired to do much, and just let him get in with us. I've noticed that he does it more when he's been to nursery than when it's school holidays, so I think he's probably just less relaxed. I'm leaving it for now, but know that at some point I need to start getting up and putting him back to bed if he comes through. I think that's going to be the only way to stop it. "*

If your child is a night-waker, firstly work on helping them to learn to self-settle (see page 36). If they call for you, go in and reassure them. Keep lights dim, and aim to be calm, quiet and even boring! Avoid eye contact, explain to them that it is still night-time and they need to stay in bed and go back to sleep. Using a repetitive phrase can be helpful such as, 'It's night-time, sleep now'.

Make sure that you are consistent about your child remaining in their own bed. Always take them back to their bed if they come in to you. Children with this issue benefit from a clear routine and clear expectations. Make sure that your child falls asleep in the place where they will wake: it can be scary and disorientating to drop off on the sofa, the buggy, the car, or in the parental bed, then wake in a different room.

Some children will respond well to a reward system with stars or stickers for staying in their own bed. You may want to start with a small reward, like a sticker in the morning for going back to their own bed during the night, if you feel staying in bed is a long way off for your child. Whether your child responds to reward charts or not, remember to praise them for staying in bed if they do.

It can take many repeats of this routine to help your child to learn to go back to sleep when it is night-time, but repeating will work eventually. If you continue to struggle, speak to a sleep specialist: see the resources section for people who can help and their contact details.

Children who rise early

Some children are just early risers: if you have a 'lark' you'll find them chatty and positive in the mornings. They might wake at the same early hour regardless of late nights, and be at their most energetic. Do not worry if this sounds like your child: many of the suggestions below will help you keep them in bed for a little longer regardless.

Children wake early for a number of reasons. Add up how long your child sleeps, including night-time and naps. If a young child needed eleven hours of sleep, and napped for two hours, that's only nine hours left for night-time sleep. If they drop off at 7 p.m., they could wake up at 4 a.m., which shows just how easy it is to go wrong! On the other hand, if that same child was woken after a forty-five-minute nap, that would leave a need for ten hours sleep at night. Put them to bed at 8 p.m., and they would wake at 6. If the child didn't nap at all, they may wake at 7. Try doing this with your own child's sleep patterns. It doesn't help to cut naps altogether in young children, but by the age of two to three you should be cutting back. If your child is older than this and still napping, experiment with what they need.

Some children will respond well to a change in bedtime. Do this gradually: make bedtime ten to fifteen minutes later for a few days, then later again. Within a week or two you will be able to tell if this is helping your child sleep in.

There are some practical tips which may also help you, and your child, get more sleep in the morning: if your child is disturbed by light or noise, if they are waking to wee or being disturbed by a dirty nappy, and if they might be hungry, look at the section on the physical causes of waking at the start of this chapter (see pages 27–29).

Nell says:

> *Delia and Kris are early wakers, while James is an owl, not a lark. Delia and Kris need less sleep in the morning, while James would always sleep in if we let him. Of course, he is the one who we struggle to get to go to bed. When Delia was a toddler I didn't realize what was going wrong: she'd be up at five every morning. I'd let her have a long nap in the middle of the day. Sometimes she napped for three hours, because she and I were both shattered. She'd be asleep at 7 p.m. routinely. Add in the fact she's never slept quite as long as the books say, and it was no wonder she was up so early. I got wise with the boys, though, and have been slightly obsessive about not letting them sleep too long at naptime. In fact, James stopped napping relatively early, but would sleep a solid twelve hours, so I put it down to the fact that he liked being awake during the day when his big sister was around, and adapted our routine accordingly.*

You may also want to check whether there are any other physical reasons for early waking – see page 27 for a reminder. If your child takes medication, this may be wearing off. They may then be woken by physical discomfort. If there is no apparent physical reason, and the measures suggested above don't help, it may be time to seek help from a sleep specialist.

Carly has tried lots of things to improve Tim's sleep, some of which have helped more than others. She says, 'To help with early waking we have installed blackout blinds. It has not solved it, but means he wakes at a slightly more reasonable hour.' Tim's sleep patterns affect the family when going on holiday. Carly says:

Being away on holiday can be a nightmare – Tim will often wake around 5 a.m. as he is excited. We camp and unfortunately canvas is no protection at all from sound, so I usually end up entertaining him for about three hours every morning as quietly as possible to avoid rousing the whole campsite. In previous years this required much advance planning and copious amounts of scrapbooking, art and craft, reading, nursery rhymes etc. These days we still do stuff together but thank god for the invention of the iPad!

If your child is an early waker look out for a sleep training clock. These clocks can be set to display sunshine when it is time to get up, and stars or a moon at bedtime, so that kids know when it's time to get up and when it isn't. The Gro-clock (available from the Gro Store – see the resources section) is good for children with SEN as it is age-appropriate even for older children and doesn't look babyish.

Also check that the curtains are thick enough, as light entering rooms in the early hours may cause some children to wake up, particularly if they are light-sensitive. See Chapter 6 for more advice.

Feeding during the night

Babies feed at night because their stomachs are too small to take in enough food to last them more than a few hours. Add in their tremendous rate of growth and you will understand why your baby needs milk every few hours round the clock. As your baby turns into a toddler, though, for most children, night feeds will stop. For a few children with special needs however, night feeding may be a necessity.

Some children need all or part of their daily nutritional requirements via a tube. There are a wide range of conditions where tube feeding can help, either temporarily or permanently. Research has shown that tube feeding can lead to disturbed or delayed sleep for the child.[5] As a parent you may also find it hard to sleep due to anxiety in case anything goes wrong. If you worry about the tube coming loose, use tape to secure the tube down your child's back and run it out through a pyjama leg. Parents have used pipe insulation to prevent the tubes from tangling. There are special sleep suits available to fit your child if they are tube fed. These are available from Rackerty's (see the resources section for contact details). If night feeds cause serious sleep issues, seek guidance from your healthcare professional about your concerns.

You may find that your child is woken by a wet bed if the feeding tube detaches. Make sure that you have a mattress cover: double layering a sheet and a mattress cover over a second sheet and a mattress cover can make it easy to remove the top layer only for fast night-time changes; or you can use a waterproof draw sheet. If your child is woken by vomiting, check that the bed is tilted adequately: gradient recommendations vary between 30 and 45% to ensure that the feed stays down. If the tube feeding continues to be an issue, discuss the option of moving the timing of the feed with your specialist. See *Food and Your Special Needs Child* for more about tube feeding.

Anxiety problems

Anxiety can keep your child up at night. This is something that can cause difficulties with dropping off to sleep. If your child is anxious, here are some tips:

✓ Create time during the day for your child to share their worries with you. This might be during the journey home from school, perhaps, if things occur at school. Make sure you ask your child if they have worries well before bedtime so you have time to help

✓ Develop a good, calming bedtime routine (see pages 31–33). In particular, avoid activities that will stimulate your child's mind

✓ Give your child a notepad where they can write down concerns that occur to them after bedtime. If your child is able to write this can be enough to get the concern out of their mind

✓ For non-writers, offer a worry doll or a small toy that they can tell their problems to. They can put the doll under their pillow, and you can tell your child that the doll will worry for them, or you may remove the doll as a symbol of the worry going away

✓ Look for ways to help your child relax, such as a local yoga class for children. Tattybumpkin and Yogabugs both offer classes across the UK, or ask at your local yoga centre. There are also training courses for teachers who would like to be able to offer yoga at school. If yoga isn't suitable, there are many recordings and books for you to read that can help your child wind down at bedtime – see www.relaxkids.com for lots of ideas

Claire says, 'We read a book at bedtime then I put music on or a relaxation CD. It works very well. I've done it since I was three months pregnant so it is a familiar sound for her.'

If anxiety is a significant problem for your child, ask your child's GP or specialist for a clinical psychology referral in order to get specialist support.

Sharing their parents bed

Many parents end up with a child in their bed for pragmatic reasons: it can be the only way that everyone gets some sleep. Other people make an active choice to bed share. If your child has additional needs, you may find that it is easier to ensure they are safe at night when you are in the same bed. However, bed sharing can cause disturbed sleep for some families.

If you would like your child to spend more of the night in their own bed, read these tips, and learn more in Chapter 7.

If your child starts the night in your bed:

✓ Start by introducing your child to the idea of sleeping in their own bed. You may entice them if you buy a new bed, or simply make sure that their bedroom is an attractive place to be

✓ Some children sleep in their own room for daytime naps: explain to your child that now they are older they could sleep in their own room at night too

✓ Make sure your child knows where you will be at night. Explain that you will be in your bed, and they will be in theirs and that you'd like them to stay there

If your child climbs into your bed during the night:

✓ Can your child self-settle? If not, they may be waking and seeking your bed for reassurance. If you don't wake when your child climbs into bed and you want to get on top of the issue, consider hanging wind chimes in your doorway or use a door alarm to wake you. See pages 35–36 in this chapter for more on teaching your child to self-settle.

For both situations:

✓ If your child comes to you at night, reassure them and return them to their bed. It should only take a few nights to build a pattern where they are used to sleeping in their own room

Summary

There are many reasons why children suffer from disturbed sleep. Start by completing the sleep diary in Chapter 1. This will help you establish whether your child's sleep issues are related to physical discomfort or behavioural issues.

Read through the list of physical issues that can disturb your child's sleep. Is your child waking because they are hot or cold, wet or soiled, hungry or thirsty? What strategies could you use to address these issues? If a physical issue such as illness or pain is a problem you may want to talk to your doctor or pharmacist.

The majority of sleep issues are behavioural. There are a few main strategies to help you improve sleep in this case. Firstly, check your bedtime routine. Make sure that your child is calm and knows that the same things will happen every evening in the run-up to bedtime. Secondly, has your child learnt to self-settle? If you need to be there for them to drop off to sleep, consider working to help your child to learn to self-settle. This will have benefits both in the evening and during the night when they enter lighter phases of sleep.

If you look at the physical and behavioural aspects of sleep, and pick strategies from this chapter to help your child, you should find that their sleep improves.

Chapter 3
Other Sleep Problems

In this chapter we explore a range of sleep problems that children may experience. We also discuss sleep problems that may have medical implications and consider when to seek advice. It is important that as a parent you are well informed about sleep issues so you can find the help that your child needs. In this chapter we hear from a number of leading practitioners and organizations and provide you with useful and up-to-date information.

If your child is displaying some unusual bedtime behaviours you should always seek the advice of a medical practitioner. Your health visitor should be contacted if your child is under the age of five. You may want to consult your school nurse if your child is over five or speak to your GP. If your child has a paediatrician be sure to tell them about the sleep issues that are concerning you as they can be a useful part of any assessment process. The paediatrician is also well placed to make appropriate referrals to ensure that your child gets access to the right professionals. Read on to find out about a range of sleep issues and see whether they fit what your child is going through.

Nightmares and night terrors

Children may experience nightmares and, less commonly, night terrors. Parents often mistake nightmares for night terrors and vice versa. In this section we will outline the differences and how to deal with each.

Nightmares

A nightmare is a frightening dream that causes a child to awaken in a state of distress; they may be worried about going back to sleep. Nightmares are common and are often related to developmental stages. For example, toddlers may start to have nightmares if they are worried about separating from their parents. Older children may develop fears of monsters and the dark which can play out in their nightmares. Sometimes nightmares may be related to things that have been seen or heard during the day but very often they may not relate to anything in particular. They are more likely to occur when a child is unwell with a raised temperature or is stressed or anxious.

Dr Heather Elphick is a sleep paediatrician at Sheffield Children's Hospital. She tells us, 'Nightmares usually happen in the second half of the night as they occur in REM sleep. The child can usually remember the dream, seeks comfort from the parent and can be consoled with reassurance. The child may, however, take a long time to fall back to sleep.'

Dr Elphick advises, 'Medical input is not usually needed for nightmares unless the child is suffering from sleep deprivation due to insomnia in the case of severe nightmares associated with anxiety or post-traumatic stress disorder. Behavioural interventions would be the most appropriate treatment.'

Emma Sweet is a sleep practitioner specializing in behavioural interventions and says:

" *It is important that children are offered reassurance if they suffer from a nightmare. Nightmares can be frightening and it may take time for them to settle back to sleep. Parents should not buy into the child's nightmare. For example, if the child says that there are monsters under the bed, searching for the monsters may actually cause the child some confusion. After all, if there aren't such things as monsters, why are my parents looking for them? Some children find a dream catcher hanging up in the room works well for them. A good bedtime routine is essential as well in setting the scene for a restful night's sleep.* "

Night terrors

Night terrors are not common: statistics suggest that only around only around 1–6% of people will experience a night terror in their lifetime. They can affect boys and girls equally and usually occur between the ages of three and twelve years old. Night terrors tend to peak around the age of three-and-a-half years and lessen during adolescence. Less than 1% of adults have night terrors.

Dr Elphick explains:

ʔʔ *Night terrors are one presentation of a group of sleep disorders known as parasomnias (partial arousal sleep disorders) that result in partial waking from sleep with associated behaviours such as screaming, kicking and thrashing, often with a look of fear and panic. The child may not recognize the parent and although appears frightened cannot be comforted. They often have no recollection of the event the next morning.* ʔʔ

Night terrors usually happen during the first few hours of the night as they occur in the transition between deep non-REM sleep and arousal from sleep at the end of the first long deep-sleep phase. Night terrors may last up to thirty minutes but you will find that your child settles quickly back to sleep after an episode.

There is a direct link between night terrors and sleep deprivation so if your child has sleep issues they may be more at risk of suffering with night terrors. Other triggers can include a high temperature, sleep apnoea, or medical conditions such as asthma or gastro-oesophageal reflux. Sometimes children begin to have night terrors following a change in their routine, such as moving into a new room or following a holiday.

Although it is distressing for parents to witness their child having a night terror, they are not thought to be harmful. You need to remember that your child is not aware of what is happening. It is important to keep calm and to not attempt to wake them. Ensure that your child doesn't hurt themselves as sometimes children start to walk around too when they have a night terror. Wait until the night terror has passed and you will find that your child quickly settles back into a restful sleep. There is no need to draw your child's attention to the fact that they had a night terror the next day as they will not be able to relate to what you are talking about which may cause them to feel confused and anxious.

While night terrors are not dangerous some parents choose to take action to try to minimize the chances of them occurring. A good sleep routine is important so that a child is well rested; paying attention to diet to eliminate any food or drink that may be causing your child to become over-stimulated in the lead-up to bedtime can be helpful too.

If your child is experiencing frequent night terrors then use a sleep diary to plot the times that they occur. It is possible to disrupt a child's sleep cycle so that they avoid a night terror. Note the times that the night terrors occur over a period of a week; if they happen at a regular time each night then you can rouse your child fifteen minutes prior to this time. You do not have to fully awaken them; the aim is to disrupt their sleep. Tucking them in may be enough to wake them partially: this can be an effective way of management. If the times that the night terrors occur are not consistent but there are physical signs that one may be approaching, such as your child kicking or moving around more in bed, you can take this as a cue for disrupting their sleep cycle. After a few nights of a parent disrupting their child's sleep cycle the night terrors usually diminish.

Using breathable bedding can also be helpful in order to ensure that your child does not get too hot. More details about bedding can be found in Chapter 6.

If you are concerned about the intensity or frequency of your child's night terrors you should seek medical advice. Dr Elphick says:

" *A medical referral is needed if there are unusual features, for example, drooling, stiffening, jerking, especially if there has been a significant head injury in the past, episodes are short and recurrent or repetitive screaming, kicking or thrashing are prominent. These features may suggest a rare form of epilepsy which may need scans and further treatment. Medical intervention may be needed for night terrors if a child is not responding to behavioural interventions and the episodes are causing significant disruption to the child and family, or if there is a fear that the child is a danger to him/herself or other family members.* 〕〕

Michelle shares with us how she found dealing with night terrors:

〔〔 *Charlie was three years old when he started to suffer with night terrors. We were just going through the assessment process for autism and my stress levels were at an all-time high. Charlie had never slept particularly well and used to wake frequently throughout the night. One night I heard the most awful scream about half an hour after he'd gone to sleep. I ran upstairs and Charlie was sitting bolt upright in bed with his eyes wide open; he looked utterly terrified. I actually looked around the room thinking he must have seen something in there. He was sweating and trembling; it was the most awful thing to witness and he seemed oblivious to me trying to comfort him. The episode went on for a few minutes and then he simply lay down and went back to sleep. I was really shaken up after witnessing it and didn't know what on earth had happened; it sounds ridiculous looking back but I even wondered if he'd seen a ghost! It happened again the next night and my husband witnessed it this time and was as distressed about it as I was. I phoned the Child Development Centre and asked to speak to a member of the assessment team and explained what had happened. The nursery nurse suggested that it was a night terror and gave me some advice about disrupting his sleep cycle by going into his room and waking him up a little. I did this and the night terrors stopped as quickly as they had started. I want to share my story as I know how frightening these can be for parents to witness and I'm just grateful that somebody was able to give me some sound advice at the time. While as parents, we were both terrified, Charlie was blissfully unaware of what had been happening in the night!* 〕〕

If you are still unsure, the following table may help you to work out whether your child is suffering with nightmares or night terrors:

	Night terror	Nightmare
Time of night it occurs	First half of the night	Second half of the night
Can your child recall the episode?	No	Yes
Can you console your child?	No	Yes
Does your child recognize you during the episode?	No	Yes
Duration	Usually 5–15 mins	May be prolonged

Sleepwalking

Sleepwalking is another form of parasomnia and is more likely to occur in children who have night terrors. Like night terrors it occurs during the transition stage between deep sleep and waking. It usually occurs after the first long period of deep sleep so is more likely to occur during the first third of the night and usually happens just once a night. It is estimated that 3–4% of children sleepwalk on a regular basis and up to 40% of us sleepwalk at least once in our lifetime. There is a family history of sleepwalking in 80% of children who sleepwalk. Sleepwalking generally begins in childhood with peak incidence between the ages of four and eight. Most children tend to outgrow it by adulthood.

Episodes of sleepwalking may last up to half an hour and may be associated with bed-wetting. Children who are sleepwalking usually move around the environment with their usual action; their eyes may be open but they remain asleep. As with night terrors, because your child is actually asleep, they will not recall the event the next morning.

Dr Elphick says:

There are a number of myths around sleepwalking such as it is people acting out their dreams and it is associated with epilepsy. Neither of these are accurate, neither does it indicate a psychological or psychiatric problem. It is not dangerous to waken someone who is sleepwalking although it is not advisable as it can lead to them lashing out due to being confused and disorientated.

While sleepwalking generally begins in childhood, nobody knows *why* it occurs. It has been suggested that it may be due to different parts of the brain developing at different rates and therefore affected children's brains do not recognize the sleep cycles as effectively as the adult brain. In addition to this, children have slower delta waves during non-REM sleep and this immaturity of the brain may be the cause of an increased tendency to sleepwalk. Another theory is that a hormone imbalance may trigger the sleepwalking, as it is during non-REM sleep that there is a release of growth hormones in children.

There may be a number of triggers for sleepwalking which include sleep deprivation and stress. A high temperature may increase the incident of sleepwalking and episodes may be triggered by other sleep disturbances such as coughing, bed-wetting or restless leg syndrome. It is thought that parasomnias may be triggered when the sleep cycle is unexpectedly disrupted.

Tips for managing sleepwalking

Here are some tips to help you manage your child's sleepwalking:

✓ Identify any potential hazards and put in place safety measures such as window locks and stair gates
✓ Disrupt the sleep cycle as described in the treatment of night terrors
✓ Do not wake your child during an episode; try to steer them back to bed to resettle
✓ Ensure that you have a good sleep routine and a calm environment to help to promote more restful sleep

Dr Elphick says:

❝ *If there are unusual or concerning repetitive actions or other features then seek medical advice. The onset of sleepwalking is usually in childhood and adults who sleepwalk have usually done so since they were a child. Onset of sleepwalking during adolescence or adulthood may be a symptom of an underlying problem and therefore should be medically assessed. A medical referral is also recommended if there are symptoms of other nocturnal medical problems such as sleep apnoea, bed-wetting, reflux and so on. If events are causing daytime tiredness due to sleep disturbance or if the child has performed acts which may be dangerous, such as opening windows or attempting to leave the house, medical guidance should be sought.* "

Rhythmic movement disorder

Some children find movement comforting and may rock back and forth in order to self-soothe. This behaviour may also appear at night-time just before they fall asleep. Although many parents share that they find the behaviour somewhat alarming, as long as the child is safe then this rhythmic movement is not harmful. Rhythmic movement disorder is often found in children with sensory issues and particularly those on the autism spectrum.

Sometimes children will engage in movements that can cause injury to themselves. Some children may make a sound while they rock. Research suggests that rhythmic movement disorder is most frequently observed in boys and serves a soothing function. Many children outgrow this kind of movement. Encouraging your child to access activities during the day that include rocking can be helpful. For example, using a rocking chair or a swing can provide them with the feedback that they require. When rocking or head-banging becomes vigorous and you are concerned about safety you should seek medical help.

Carol has three children with autism and the youngest has rhythmic movement disorder.

" *I was really worried about Hope because she rocks herself to sleep quite vigorously every night. If she wakes in the night then the rocking will start again. It looks unusual and far from comforting. I went to a sleep workshop and the sleep practitioner explained about rhythmic movement disorder. It really helped to get a name for the behaviours that I was seeing and I felt reassured that it wasn't a problem and just her way of soothing herself to sleep.* "

Restless legs syndrome

Children with additional needs may find it difficult to communicate to us what difficulties they are experiencing. A young man with additional needs and restless leg syndrome drew a picture of spiders running up and down his legs, which helped his care team to form a diagnosis of restless legs syndrome.

Sufferers describe the sensation as a feeling of crawling beneath the skin which is unpleasant and leads them to want to continually move their legs. The condition is most prevalent in middle age but can occur in childhood. If you suspect that your child has restless legs syndrome it would be worth mentioning to your GP as in some cases it can indicate an iron deficiency and can be resolved effectively. Massaging legs may also be recommended alongside a warm bath.

Bruxism

Bruxism, or teeth grinding as it is more commonly called, can disrupt children's sleep patterns. If left untreated it can cause dental issues, headaches and aching of the jaw. Research suggests that children who grind their teeth in their sleep are more likely to be hyperactive and have behavioural issues; there is a strong link between bruxism and Attention Deficit Hyperactivity Disorder (ADHD). Episodes of teeth grinding can last just a few seconds but may occur numerous times each hour. If you are worried about your child's teeth grinding you can contact the Bruxism Association who have a website and a dedicated helpline www.bruxism.org.uk.

Sleep apnoea

Sleep apnoea is a condition where breathing pauses during sleep. This can lead to a drop in oxygen levels or a disturbance in sleep. The British Lung Foundation states that, 'Obstructive sleep apnoea is quite common and may affect up to 1 in 30 children. It affects boys and girls equally.' There is more than one type of sleep apnoea.

Kath Hope runs an organization called Hope2Sleep and aims to raise awareness of sleep apnoea and provide support for existing sufferers and their families. Kath has sleep apnoea herself. She is a member of the British Lung Foundation's Advisory Panel and Expert Patient to Guy's & St Thomas' Sleep Disorders Centre. Kath tells us, 'Sleep apnoea is vastly under-diagnosed and it is estimated that around 80% of people living with sleep apnoea are undiagnosed at present. Sleep apnoea was initially thought to be mainly just present in overweight men with large neck collars, but medics now realize that this is not true and it can affect anyone, including children.'

The good news for children is that many people can be cured of sleep apnoea by the removal of their tonsils and/or adenoids. There are two types of sleep apnoea. Read on to find out more.

Central Sleep Apnoea (CSA)

This occurs when the signals from the brain fail to send messages to the muscles and the child 'forgets' to breathe. This most commonly occurs in children with neuro-disabilities or underlying neurological problems, or in premature babies. The parent will notice a quiet pause in breathing, followed by the child quietly starting to breathe normally again. If there is blueness around the lips or you are concerned about your child's breathing while they are asleep, seek medical advice.

Obstructive Sleep Apnoea (OSA)

This happens when there is an obstruction to breathing within the airway. In children this is usually due to enlarged tonsils and/or adenoids and may be made worse by floppiness of the airway tissues. Dr Heather Elphick says:

Airway floppiness may occur in typically developing children but is often associated with neurodevelopmental or muscular problems or some syndromes, including Down's syndrome. Obstructive Sleep Apnoea may be caused by obesity, disorders of facial structure or severe gastro-oesophageal reflux, but the vast majority of cases are in typically developing, otherwise well children who have enlarged tonsils or adenoids and respond well to surgery to remove these.

For children with Down's syndrome, sleep apnoea can be extremely common. Research suggests around 45% of children with Down's syndrome will suffer from Obstructive Sleep Apnoea. This can be due to enlarged tonsils, the facial structure of the child and low tone of the muscles in the upper airway.

With OSA the child's breathing may be associated with snoring followed by a pause in breathing; sometimes this ends with a loud snort. The chest may be moving up and down more than usual and sufferers can look as though they are struggling to breathe. They may wake briefly and change position to try to relieve the apnoea. In the morning the child may be difficult to wake due to a disturbed night's sleep. Medical assessment should again be sought immediately if there is any blueness around the lips. Medical evaluation will include an assessment of any underlying medical conditions, an examination of the tonsils and possibly an assessment of oxygen levels during sleep.

SYMPTOMS OF SLEEP APNOEA

Common symptoms of sleep apnoea include snoring, although this is also fairly common in children who do not have sleep apnoea! Pauses in breath noticed by parents, followed by a gasp or a snort, are another common symptom. Some children may adopt unusual sleeping positions such as sleeping with their head bent backwards, others may be restless and wake frequently. Unusual noises such as choking sounds, snorts or gasps may be heard while the child is asleep. Open mouthed breathing may be observed as can bed-wetting, although again this is common and may be unrelated to sleep apnoea, as we will discuss later in this chapter.

Children with sleep apnoea can also present with symptoms during the daytime. Sleep deprivation may lead their behaviour to change and they may become more irritable or even hyperactive. Concentration levels may decrease and performance at school may be affected. You may notice breathing through the mouth during the day and nasal-sounding speech; some children have difficulties swallowing. General health can also be impaired; a child with disrupted sleep may have growth or weight issues. They may experience early-morning headaches or pick up illnesses more often than their peers.

Dr Elphick tells us, 'The parent's main fear is that the child may stop breathing, but the medical concerns are the long-term consequences of low oxygen levels which can lead to heart strain and failure to grow properly. There are also educational and behavioural problems associated with sleep disturbance.'

TREATMENT OF SLEEP APNOEA

It is important that sleep apnoea is treated. Kath Hope tells us, 'Sleep apnoea can be a serious condition due to its links with other life-threatening illness and must be treated. Not only will this lower the risk of other linked medical conditions, but general physical and mental health, along with increased energy levels, will improve.'

CPAP (Continuous Positive Airways Pressure) may also be used. This is where the sufferer wears a mask and the air from the machine prevents the airways from collapsing. There are a number of variations of this machine and sleep clinicians can assess your child to determine the most appropriate.

For some youngsters removal of the tonsils and/or adenoids can cure sleep apnoea although symptoms may return during adulthood. A Mandibular Advancement Device (MAD) can be used in mild cases of sleep apnoea. This is an oral device which is made by an orthodontist or dentist to be worn during sleep. It is designed to bring the tongue and lower jaw forward.

For more information about sleep apnoea visit Kath's website www.hope2sleepguide.co.uk.

If you are at all concerned about your child's breathing during their sleep seek advice from your GP immediately.

Bed-wetting or enuresis

Bed-wetting, or enuresis as you may hear it referred to, can be a common issue for youngsters with additional needs. Eileen Jacques is the information and helpline manager from ERIC (Education and Resources for Improving Childhood Continence), the only national children's charity dedicated to supporting children, young people and their families with wetting and soiling problems.

ERIC offers practical ideas, information and resources to help manage or overcome the difficulties associated with bed-wetting, including a confidential helpline, email support and a text messaging service. ERIC also provides an online message board for parents and children and a website with lots of valuable information to download free of charge. For more information visit the website at www.eric.org.uk.

Some children may grow out of bed-wetting yet for many the issue continues into adulthood. For parents, bed-wetting can be difficult to cope with. Rachel's daughter is thirteen years old, has learning difficulties and still wets the bed frequently.

I use pads at night for Chelsea to try to keep her as comfortable as possible but as she is getting older she seems to produce more urine. She will frequently wake up in the night soaking wet. I find it incredibly frustrating as I'm tired and the last thing I want to be doing is changing her and then changing her bed. I've found that some mattress protectors are definitely more effective than others. I think it's a case of experimenting until you find a product that you are happy with. I now use duvet protectors and find these brilliant. I look for breathable products too so that she doesn't get overheated in bed.

Eileen Jacques says, 'We don't fully understand why some children take longer than others to master the art of staying dry, but we know that it is not linked to poor toilet training or laziness on the child's part. It does tend to go in families and there is a hereditary factor.'

As bed-wetting occurs during sleep, the child has no conscious control over it and is even unaware that it is happening. Eileen says:

A lack of the right levels of the natural hormone vasopressin, which causes the kidneys to concentrate urine production at night, has been shown to cause bed-wetting. This means that rather than a reduced amount of urine being produced overnight, the kidneys produce daytime amounts of urine and the bladder cannot hold it. Indications that night-time vasopressin is lacking include large, wet patches of urine in the night and wetting soon after sleep, in the early part of the night. Medication to replace the inadequate hormone can be prescribed. "

Another reason that bed-wetting may occur is an overactive bladder. Eileen explains:

" *The muscles of an overactive bladder contract before the bladder is full and this signals that it needs to empty urgently. Signs of an overactive bladder will sometimes be apparent during the day with the child needing to go to the toilet often and very urgently and they may have damp pants during the day. At night the child will often have small wet patches in the bed and wake up after wetting. Medication can be prescribed to relax the strong signals from the bladder.* "

The third and final reason that bed-wetting may occur is that the child doesn't receive the signal sent from the bladder to the brain which tells them to wake up and empty their bladder. Eileen says, 'Bed-wetting alarms can be useful in these cases but need the child to be motivated and want to use one and have good support from their carers. Alarms help a child to learn to hold their urine at night and so can help with a permanent cure as the child learns the skill'.

If you do need to change your child during the night, keep the lights low so as not to interfere with melatonin production. Do not engage in conversation other than to offer reassurance.

Other factors around bed-wetting may include constipation and urinary tract infections. If your child is dry during the daytime but consistently wetting at night-time it is important to get them checked by your GP or a health professional.

Epilepsy

The relationship between epilepsy and sleep can be a complex one. Epilepsy can be mistaken for a sleep disorder and vice versa. Sleep disorders can make the epilepsy worse and epilepsy can worsen sleep disorders. Research has found that children with epilepsy are more at risk of having a poor quality sleep which is of shorter duration. There are many different types of epilepsy, some of which occur during the night. If you are concerned that epilepsy may be impacting on your child's sleep, medical advice should be sought. If a child is having seizures during their sleep it can affect their whole night's sleep. Sleep patterns can become much lighter following a seizure and REM sleep may disappear altogether. Epilepsy Action supports people with epilepsy in various different ways including via a free-phone helpline, email support and an online community. You can find their website by logging on to www.epilepsy.org.uk.

Medication and sleep

Some medications have unwanted side effects that can impact on your child's sleep quality. Some epilepsy medications, for example, are linked to sleep issues and may trigger night terrors. If your child is taking medication and has sleep issues it would be worth checking with a medical practitioner whether any of the sleep problems that you are dealing with are linked with the medication and, if so, whether there are any alternatives for your child to try.

Some children need to take medication during the night, like Sonia's son, who has complex medical needs. She tells us:

I used to wake Tom for his medicine when I came to bed but found he had trouble settling back to sleep. I've now taken some tips that I've received from The Children's Sleep Charity and made a few changes. I changed the lightbulb for a start in the night light and replaced the bright white bulb with a glowing orange bulb. This has made a signifi-cant difference as I'm able to see what I'm doing, which is incredibly important when administering medication, but Tom doesn't seem to wake fully like he did with the brighter light. I also kept a sleep diary so that I could work out Tom's sleep cycles and I can go in and give the medication when he is at a point of partial awakening. This is much easier than trying to rouse him from a deep sleep. Since I've imple-mented the changes I've found that he settles back to sleep far more quickly and the night wakings that used to follow have reduced as well. 𝟻𝟻

Read more about medication and sleep in Chapter 4.

Pain management

If your child is in pain during the night then their sleep patterns will become disturbed. It is important to try to identify what may be causing the pain so that strategies can be put in place to try to alleviate/manage the pain more effectively. For some children the pain may be due to leg spasms or postural issues. If you suspect this is the case it is important to liaise with the physiotherapists and occupational therapists involved in your child's care.

Sharing information with practitioners

Sometimes it is necessary to share information around your child's sleep with practitioners involved in their care. This can help you to look at the sleep issue from a different perspective and it may be that professional intervention is required. If you are at all concerned about your child's sleep issues then do seek medical help.

When attending appointments it is important that you feel prepared and that you manage to get across all the information that you wish to share.

Sharing information tips

Here are some tips to help you to communicate any problems effectively to the relevant professionals:

✓ Spend some time writing down all the issues that are concerning you about your child's sleep
✓ Include information about how your child's sleep issues impact on their daytime behaviour
✓ State how it is affecting you as a family and your relationships
✓ Take two weeks' worth of completed sleep diaries if possible to show clearly the sleep patterns that you are dealing with

✓ If your child engages in unusual sleep behaviours take a recording of these so that you can show the practitioners exactly what you are talking about

✓ If the professional that you are sharing the information with is unable to help you ask them to refer you to somebody who can help

✓ Write down a list of questions that you would like answered about the sleep issues

✓ Don't be afraid to take out your list during the appointment to jog your memory

✓ Ask for a contact number so that you can ring back if you have any further questions once you have left the appointment

Summary

There are many issues that can impact and disrupt a child's sleep, and that of their parent or family. In this chapter we have explored some of the medical reasons why children may have sleep issues. We have also explored parasomnias and simple methods to manage these more effectively. If your child's sleep problem is impacting on you or them in a significant way it is important to approach a practitioner or an organization such as The Children's Sleep Charity, as they can signpost you towards further help.

Chapter 4
Daytime Activity and Sleep

Have you noticed that your child's sleep is affected by the things you do during the day? It can be easy to see the link between an exciting day and difficulty dropping off to sleep, but there are other links between daytime activity and sleep too. This chapter will help you look at how your child's activities may affect their sleep. In particular, we focus on food and diet and their relationship to sleep. You can also find out about how exercise can improve sleep. Finally, the chapter looks in more depth at medication and how it can affect sleep.

Remember to complete the sleep diary from Chapter 1 as this will help you identify daytime events that might be impairing your child's sleep, and if you think that food may affect your child's sleep after reading more, link this in with ideas for the food diary later in this chapter.

Vicki says:

David was a nightmare with diet and sleep. He was very active during the day and he'd never been a particularly good sleeper. He never slept well, to be honest. He was always on the go, didn't nap when he should have. He had difficulties settling and staying asleep, and woke early! My mum commented on his behaviour after she gave him a chocolate biscuit; he very quickly became very active and couldn't settle to do anything. I noticed that chocolate was definitely a trigger for his hyperactivity and did my best to avoid it. He used to love fresh orange juice to drink and had lots of it! I thought that I was being a good mum by giving him something so natural. What I'd not realized however is that it is full of natural sugar and it was giving him an energy rush too. Once I eliminated it from his diet he was much calmer in himself.

Diet and how it impacts on sleep

What you eat and drink can affect your sleep. Look at your child during the day: how do they behave when they are hungry? Thinking of yourself for a moment, how do you feel when you are trying to concentrate on something just before lunch? And how does your child behave when they have just had a big piece of cake? Remember your last Christmas meal where you ate far too much? How did you feel then?

Food is designed to energize you and lack of food, or even lack of the correct food, can cause behaviour problems. Digesting food takes energy too: all this can affect how your child sleeps. Very simply, eating too much or too little can disrupt sleep. If you have ever been hungry at bedtime, you may recognize how it makes it harder to drop off to sleep. A snack at bedtime can help some people sleep, but too much food can cause digestive discomfort that leads to wakefulness.

Sleep is controlled by a range of chemicals in the body, and scientists have studied the role of diet in supplying what your body needs to make the chemicals that promote a good night's sleep. Research is still continuing in this vein: there remain areas of uncertainty and conflicting evidence. Read on to find out what is known, and consider how diet might be affecting your child's sleep.

Caffeine

Caffeine is a definite cause of insomnia, as it is a stimulant. Most parents wouldn't let their children drink tea or coffee at a young age. However, you may not know that caffeine is also contained in chocolate and cola drinks. Plus, the energy drinks that are increasingly popular with teens also contain caffeine. If your child has sleep problems, cut out chocolate, cocoa and cola drinks and, for older children, avoid tea, coffee or energy drinks.

Some medications also contain caffeine. Read the label or ask the pharmacist whether your child's medication may affect their sleep.

Sugar

Have you noticed whether your child's sleep is affected when they eat cakes, biscuits or sweets? Some children are more sensitive to sugar than others. You may already know that your child becomes hyperactive after eating sweets, for example. Other children may suffer from irritability, either on eating sweet foods or a while later after the sugar is digested. Sugary snacks before bedtime can provide your child with a surge of energy which makes it hard for them to calm down and go to sleep. Your child may also wake in the night when their blood sugar drops again.

If your child usually has something sweet in the evening, try replacing it with a plainer snack: see pages 67–68 for some suggestions for foods that may help the body relax.

From indigestion to intolerance

A large meal before bed can make it hard for your child to drop off to sleep for a number of reasons. We have already mentioned that sweet snacks at this time can lead to an energy surge. If your child's digestive system is working while they sleep, they may then wake needing to empty their bowels. A big drink at bedtime may mean that your child then wakes needing to empty their bladder. Allow an hour or so between the last meal and drink of the day and bedtime.

Some foods are harder to digest than others: if your child suffers from reflux, for example, be careful what they eat before bed. Lying down will worsen the symptoms of indigestion.

Food intolerances can also contribute to insomnia. As an example, let's consider dairy products. Some studies have linked dairy intolerance to insomnia. In certain individuals dairy products can cause excess mucus production which may contribute to snoring. On the other hand, dairy foods are a good source of L-tryptophan which contributes to the creation of melatonin. This is the basis of the idea of having a milky drink before bedtime. In one study on 13-month-old infants with disturbed sleep, cow's milk intolerance was suggested as a possible cause. Removal of milk products cut the number of night wakings within five weeks. Reintroducing milk products brought the night wakings back again. However, do not remove milk products from your child's diet without consulting a doctor to discuss all the symptoms of intolerance.

See *Food and Your Special Need Child* for more on food allergies and intolerance.

Diet, sleep and specific conditions

Diet can play a role in treatment for children with specific health conditions, and this can also interact with sleep. One study looked at sleep in children who were consuming a ketogenic diet (a high fat, low carbohydrate and low protein diet) to improve their epilepsy. Seizure frequency went down, and the children spent more time in REM (dreaming) sleep.[6]

Sleep disturbances are common in children with Attention Deficit Hyperactivity Disorder (ADHD). One study looked at interrelationships between diet, sleep and behaviour in eighty-eight Australian children, aged six to thirteen years, who had been diagnosed with ADHD. Of all the children in the study, 30% had sleep disturbance. Parents who reported more sleep disturbance also reported a higher intake of carbohydrate, fats, and, most particularly, sugar. The researchers suggest that further investigation is needed in this area.[7] Another study looked at the effects of an elimination diet on physical and sleep complaints in twenty-seven children (from just under four to eight-and-a-half years of age) with ADHD. The diet group followed a five-week elimination diet; the control group adhered to their normal diet. Parents of both groups had to keep an extended diary and had to monitor the behaviour and the physical and sleep complaints of their child conscientiously. The number of physical and sleep complaints was significantly decreased in the diet group compared to the control group, with a reduction in the diet group of 77% and in the control group of 17%. Again, the researchers advise that more research is needed.[8]

Food additives and hyperactivity

As part of this section on food and sleep, you may have concerns about the effect of food additives on your child. Some food colourings have been linked to hyperactivity.[9] [10] Hyperactivity is when 'a child is overactive, cannot concentrate and acts on sudden wishes without thinking about alternatives'. Hyperactivity can make it hard for your child to learn to wind down before bed. According to the NHS, there is no single test for diagnosing hyperactivity, and experts think it affects 2–5% of children in the UK. There are other factors that influence hyperactivity in addition to additives. These include premature birth, genetics and upbringing (such as parental warmth and understanding, attitudes to punishment and over-protection amongst many other factors).

According to the NHS, if your child shows signs of hyperactivity eliminating some colours from their diet might have beneficial effects on their behaviour. These colours are used in foods including cakes, sweets, ice cream and soft drinks:

- ✓ Sunset yellow (E110)
- ✓ Quinoline yellow (E104)
- ✓ Carmoisine (E122)
- ✓ Allura red (E129)
- ✓ Tartrazine (E102)
- ✓ Ponceau 4R (E124)

Foods containing these colours must list them within the ingredients, and use the specific warning that the colour 'may have an adverse effect on activity and attention in children'. Talk to your child's healthcare provider about their behaviour and seek advice before changing their diet.[11]

The Food Standards Agency is encouraging manufacturers to find alternatives to these colours. Some manufacturers and retailers have already taken action to remove them.

Parents have also reported side effects from other additives. Emma says:

" *Annatto E160(b) definitely affects my eldest. It makes it hard to get him to bed; it affects his appetite and his temper. We discovered this when he was approximately nine months old. We changed some of our staple products and he improved within a week.*

At nine months old he was already a high needs baby. His Daddy introduced ice cream cornets as a treat, and he gradually ate his way through the whole box. He started to go to sleep later and wake up earlier, be more fussy breastfeeding, have more tantrums. It was when I took him away for a week to my mum's, without the cornets, that his sleep and feeding and temper got better. On return home, Daddy greeted him with the cornets and the boy stayed awake till 4 a.m. that night. I looked at the ingredients on the box. Everything seemed innocent, annatto is a natural colour, but I Googled it and up pops a warning that it could cause aggression and disruption in sleep patterns. We checked our cupboards and stopped using a butter-substitute spread, and started using real butter. We stopped buying orange cheese and bought white cheddar instead. I checked everything I bought and avoided annatto. We also avoid cordials with preservatives in and use organic ones now or fresh juice. It helps but now he's nine I do let things slide a bit. I also have three other boys; I have no idea if they react in the same way or not, I don't want to try and see. My eldest is currently being assessed for autism spectrum disorders and I've asked for sensitivity tests. "

Foods thought to improve sleep

As the final part of this section on food and sleep, here is some information about foods that are thought to improve sleep.

Calcium is known to help the synthesis of serotonin (the chemical that induces feelings of well-being) and enhance relaxation. Serotonin is a natural sedative. Low levels of calcium can cause nervousness and irritability.

Calcium is found in:

- ✓ Broccoli
- ✓ Carob
- ✓ Cheese
- ✓ Milk
- ✓ Spinach
- ✓ Sunflower seeds
- ✓ Yoghurt

Tryptophan is a natural dietary sleep inducer. An essential amino acid, it helps to increase the amount of serotonin in the brain. Carbohydrates help tryptophan enter the brain.

Tryptophan is found in:

✓ Chicken
✓ Soy beans
✓ Tuna
✓ Turkey
✓ Milk

B vitamins are necessary to produce serotonin from tryptophan. The vitamins needed for the generation of serotonin include B-1 or thiamine, B-3 or niacin, B-6 or pyridoxine and B-9 or folate. Foods rich in B vitamins include:

✓ Whole grains
✓ Legumes
✓ Offal
✓ Raw nuts and seeds
✓ Mushrooms
✓ Deep-sea fish
✓ Eggs
✓ Meat
✓ Dark-green vegetables

Magnesium is also part of the process. To boost magnesium in your child's diet, include some of the following:

✓ Avocados
✓ Bananas
✓ Beans
✓ Garlic
✓ Green leafy vegetables
✓ Nuts
✓ Prunes, raisins and dates
✓ Pulses
✓ Rye
✓ Wild rice
✓ Sunflower seeds
✓ Whole grains

Healthy food and drink for sleep – tips

If you want to help your child sleep better, why not give them a bedtime snack that might contain nutrients to aid sleep? Here are some tips to help you:

✓ Buy healthy foods and snacks rather than buying junk food
✓ Avoid sugary snacks which give your child a sugar high followed by a low
✓ Opt for more complex carbohydrates – whole grains and raw fruits and vegetables – which take longer to digest and avoid highs and lows
✓ Give your child their main meal well before bedtime if they seem to have lots of energy after eating. Include chicken, turkey or tuna in this meal to give your child's levels of tryptophan a boost
✓ Ensure your child does not go to bed hungry
✓ Give your child a small snack containing carbohydrates thirty minutes before bed to help metabolise the tryptophan. Try wholegrain cereal and milk, porridge, a small peanut-butter sandwich or oat biscuits and milk
✓ Make sure your child drinks milk or water rather than juice or fizzy drinks before bedtime. Some drinks or snacks may have an impact on a child's bedtime routine, and drinks with colouring or sweeteners can affect settling. Blackcurrant juice should be avoided as it can irritate the bladder and cause children to urinate more frequently

Food diaries

In Chapter 1 you read about the benefits of filling in a sleep diary to help you identify what helps your child sleep and what disrupts sleep. If, now you have read more about food and sleep, you suspect food may be affecting your child, you could consider creating a food diary.

In a food diary you need to note down everything your child eats and drinks. You can expand the food part of the sleep diary in Chapter 1, or use a stand-alone food/sleep diary as shown on the following pages.

What follows is an example of how one family completed their diary.

Child's Name: Jamie	Date: 7-14 June	Child's DOB: 2 March 2005	
	DAY 1	DAY 2	DAY 3
Breakfast – 7 a.m.	1 bowl chocolate hoops cereal	1 bowl sugar puffs	1 bowl chocolate hoops cereal
Drink	Orange juice, one cup	Orange juice, one cup	Orange juice, one cup
Morning snacks – 10.30 a.m.	1 chocolate digestive biscuit	2 custard cream biscuits	2 digestive biscuits
Drink	Glass of fruit squash	Glass of fruit squash	Glass of fruit squash
Lunch – 12 p.m.	School lunch: pizza, chocolate pudding	School lunch: fish pie, sponge pudding	School lunch: spaghetti bolognese, yoghurt
Drink	Water	Water	Water
Afternoon snacks (on the way home from school)	Crisps	Chocolate bar	Chocolate buttons
Drink	Can of lemonade	Can of cola	Can of lemonade
Dinner – 6 p.m.	Chicken nuggets and chips, chocolate mousse	Macaroni cheese, chocolate mousse	Fish fingers, potatoes and peas, chocolate mousse
Drink	Glass of cola drink	Glass of cola drink	Glass of cola drink
Evening snacks	None	None	None
Drink	Water	Water	Water
Time my child was in bed	8 p.m.	8 p.m.	8 p.m.
How my child settled	Was awake for a couple of hours in bedroom. Came down three times, asking for water, and used the toilet	Stayed awake for a couple of hours in her bedroom. Called down three times, but stayed in her room apart from using the toilet	Was awake for 1 hour in bedroom. Came down twice, asked for water, and used the toilet
Time my child went to sleep	10 p.m.	10 p.m.	9 p.m.
Night wakings	None	None	None
When my child woke in the morning	Had to wake her at 7 a.m.	Had to wake her at 7 a.m.	Had to wake her at 7 a.m.
Total hours slept	9	9	10

DAY 4	DAY 5	DAY 6	DAY 7
1 bowl chocolate hoops cereal	1 bowl sugar puffs	1 bowl chocolate hoops cereal	1 bowl sugar puffs
Orange juice, one cup	Orange juice, one cup	Orange juice, one cup	Orange juice, one cup
2 party rings	2 chocolate fingers	None	None
Glass of fruit squash	Glass of fruit squash	Glass of cola drink	Glass of cola drink
School lunch: shepherd's pie, chocolate cake	School lunch: sausage and chips, fruit	Fish and chips	Roast chicken, potatoes, carrots
Water	Water	Can of cola drink	Glass of cola drink
Crisps	Chocolate bar	None	None
Can of cola	Can of cola	None	None
Burger in a bun, chocolate mousse	Egg and chips, chocolate mousse	Pizza, chocolate mousse	Ham sandwich, chocolate mousse
Glass of cola drink	Glass of cola drink	Glass of cola drink	Glass of cola drink
None	None	None	None
Water	Water	Water	Water
8 p.m.	9 p.m.	10 p.m.	8.30 p.m.
Went to sleep quite quickly. Swimming today, which makes her tired	Stayed up with us until 9 p.m. – we took her up when she was really sleepy	Fell asleep on the sofa	Really didn't want to go to bed, screamed and cried. Crashed around in her bedroom for quite some time
8.30 p.m.	9.15 p.m.	10 p.m. approx.	10 p.m.
Wet the bed at 2 a.m.	None	None	None
Had to wake her at 7 a.m.	Had to wake her at 7 a.m.	9 a.m.	9 a.m.
10	9.45	11	11

Here is a blank template. You can copy this diary, or browse the internet for 'printable child food diary' and you will find lots of variations.

Child's Name:	Date:		Child's DOB:
	DAY 1	DAY 2	DAY 3
Breakfast			
Drink			
Morning snacks			
Drink			
Lunch			
Drink			
Afternoon snacks			
Drink			
Dinner			
Drink			
Evening snacks			
Drink			
Time my child was in bed			
How my child settled			
Time my child went to sleep			
Night wakings			
When my child woke in the morning			
Total hours slept			

DAY 4	DAY 5	DAY 6	DAY 7

Tips for using a food diary

✓ Print your diary out and pin it up near the kitchen or dining table. A quick note of what your child eats at the time they eat it will be more accurate than trying to remember later

✓ If your child eats school meals, ask the school for the menu. You may also need to ask about what they get to drink

✓ If your child is old enough you could get them involved by drawing or sticking on pictures of what they have eaten

Making changes

Once you have created your food diary, here are some suggestions that will help you test out changes that could help your child sleep:

✓ Swap sugary snacks for foods that your child can digest more slowly, and which provide less of a sugar rush

✓ Change sugary soft drinks for milk or water

✓ Change the time of your child's last meal so they have time to digest before bedtime

✓ If it looks like one food or group of foods affects your child's behaviour, talk to the GP about a referral to a dietician.

✓ Don't eliminate whole food groups from your child's diet without professional advice as this can affect their growth and development

Exercise and sleep

How much exercise does your child get? Exercise is generally thought to help your child sleep,[12] but some sorts of exercise will help more than others. One study looked at eleven healthy children aged around twelve years and compared moderate-intensity exercise with high-intensity exercise. Only high-intensity exercise resulted in better slow-wave sleep.[13] So, for some children aerobic exercise, which raises the heart rate, may have positive effects on the different chemicals in the body that contribute to sleep.

There are different benefits to other sorts of exercise too. If your child is a live wire, you could think about exercise as a way to teach them to relax. Look for a local child yoga class – see Chapter 2 for more on yoga and Chapter 8 for more on relaxation.

Another thing to consider is when your child exercises. Afternoon and early evening exercise can help your child sleep. Exercise stimulates your child's heart, muscles and brain, and raises their body temperature. Their body temperature then falls naturally as they are getting ready for bed which can help them drop off. One note of caution: vigorous exercise in the hours immediately before bed can make it harder to fall asleep.

If your child has physical impairments that make it hard for them to exercise ask their specialist for advice. You may find that a physiotherapist can put you in touch with specialist classes with activities that will suit your child.

Naps and sleep

Does your child nap? Remember that your child has a total for the number of hours they sleep during the day *and* night. Daytime naps will reduce the need for night-time sleep. See Chapter 1 for more on napping and the hours of sleep needed.

Daylight and sleep

Exposure to light in the morning helps us all wake up, but some research has shown that morning light also helps you go to sleep. It acts by regulating the biological clock: exposure to light every morning 'sets your clock' for the day. The body is most responsive to sunlight between 6 and 8.30 a.m. Direct outdoor sunlight for around thirty minutes has the most effect, while indoor lighting has little effect. If your child doesn't seem to have a strong internal body clock, try some outdoor play first thing, or walking to school if you can.

Switching off at night

If your child has problems dropping off to sleep, remember that their daytime activities can affect this. TV and computers affect how your child sleeps. One study has found that computer game playing results in significantly reduced amounts of slow-wave sleep as well as significant declines in verbal memory performance. Detrimental effects on sleep were also detected after previous computer game consumption.

Television viewing reduced sleep efficiency significantly but did not affect sleep patterns.[14]

If your child is used to watching TV in their bedroom, test out using a story CD instead. Light from the TV can hinder the body's efforts to produce melatonin, which aids sleep. Similarly, have a cut-off point for computer use: perhaps allow your child to use computer games or the computer before the evening meal, then get them to read or play board games after dinner. Try this for a week, add the results to your sleep diary and see if it helps them drop off.

Feeding at night

If your child is tube fed you may find that this can disturb their sleep. It can be the actual feeding, or discomfort from digestive processes that wakes them. Sometimes tubes leak, which can leave your child with wet clothes that wake them.

Talk to your specialist for advice on positioning. Raising the bed head can help your child's digestive function.

If your child wakes at night because they continue to urinate due to feeding, look for nappy doublers which you can add in to increase the absorbency. There are also cloth nappies specifically designed with extra absorbency for tube-fed children.

If your child's tube leaks, speak to your specialist about the fit of the tube and ask for advice on securing the tubes at night.

Medication – how it may affect sleep

Does your child take medication regularly or occasionally? Some medications can stimulate your child and stop them sleeping. For example, drugs used to treat ADHD, anti-depressants, corticosteroids and anti-convulsants can cause insomnia.

Stimulants and sleep

Pharmacist Sarah Newbury says:

❝ *As we have seen, some medications can indeed prevent sleep. Medications such as methylphenidate are actually classed as stimulants but, strangely, work to neutralize over-activity in children with ADHD. This stimulant effect is used as a benefit in this instance but presents a problematic side effect when sleep is required – as in the case of certain corticosteroids and anti-depressants. For this reason, it is often recommended that these medications be taken early on in the day where appropriate to minimize sleep disturbance. Formulation type can also be considered since modified or slow-release preparations may help to provide steadier, more uniform dosing throughout the day. A disrupted night's sleep will often lead to a disruption in daytime functioning, leaving the patient feeling tired and irritable which, in turn, makes concentrating difficult and general behaviour unpredictable.* "

If you are concerned about this – perhaps your child has started a new medication and you have seen their sleep worsen – talk to your pharmacist. They may suggest changing the time of day that your child takes the medication. If it is enough of a problem to warrant stopping the medication, do talk to your child's specialist before taking action. Never stop prescription medications without speaking to a professional first.

Depression and sleep

Depression can cause disturbed sleep in children. If your child is being assessed for depression, consider whether this may be playing a role in sleep disturbances. Although anti-depressants may make your child more upbeat during the day they can sometimes also help improve sleep quality at night. Confusingly, some anti-depressants can also make sleep worse, so again discuss what time of day is best to take the anti-depressants with the prescribing doctor or pharmacist. A tablet that causes problems when taken at night may be fine if taken earlier in the day. There are many different types of anti-depressant, and they will have different effects on sleep, so if you feel your child's medication is adversely affecting their sleep, discuss this with a professional. Do not stop the anti-depressants suddenly.

Medication to aid sleep

Some children may be prescribed medication to help them sleep. Sarah Newbury explains:

❝ *Little data exists about the safety and effectiveness of pharmacotherapy for the treatment of insomnia and other sleep disorders in children and the evidence base is often extrapolated from adult trials. However, treatment of insomnia symptoms on prescription is common, especially for children with special needs and co-morbid psychiatric disorders. Indeed, one thought is that the earlier treatment is given, the better in order that bad habits don't set in.* ❞

Sarah says:

❝ *The British National Formulary for Children (BNFC) lists sedative antihistamines and melatonin under its hypnotics section. Sedating antihistamines may cause 'hangover symptoms' during the day and have to be used with caution in epilepsy. Promethazine is a long-acting antihistamine which can be used in children over two years for insomnia but, as usual, care must be taken if taking other medications (e.g. paracetamol).* ❞

Antihistamines are often the first medications used for insomnia due to their having drowsiness as a side effect. When given to a child shortly before bedtime, they can help the child stay asleep.[15] Sarah Newbury says:

❝ *Antihistamines can be used to aid sleep but it is generally not a good idea to use a drug for its side effect, rather than its therapeutic effect. If it is necessary, then short-term use should be encouraged alongside a relaxing bedtime routine, since long-term use can result in the development of tolerance to the effects. A doctor should always be consulted.* ❞

Do not be tempted to use over-the-counter antihistamines or any other non-prescribed medications to assist your child's sleep. Seek medical advice first. Sarah Newbury stresses:

❝ *Use of over-the-counter (OTC) medications for sleep disorders is not advisable in children, largely because age restrictions and medicine product licences prevent it. In fact, the children's cough and cold formulations that once contained pseudoephedrine (decongestant) and diphenhydramine (antihistamine) have been re-formulated and are no longer available for children under the age of six years.[16] Another consideration, especially with children taking antidepressants or anti-epileptics, is possible drug interactions.* ❞

Melatonin is a hormone that is naturally produced by our bodies. It plays a critical role in the sleep cycle. Artificial melatonin medication can be effective for treating insomnia in children with physical or learning disabilities as it can help adjust the body's internal clock. Darkness should cause your child's body to produce more melatonin, which then sends signals to the body to prepare for sleep. In the morning, light should decrease melatonin production and send your child's body the signal to wake. Some people who have trouble sleeping are thought to have low levels of melatonin. It is thought that adding melatonin from supplements might help them sleep. Melatonin needs to be given shortly before bedtime and some research indicates that it can help children go to sleep. Sarah Newbury advises:

❝ *Melatonin has been widely used in doses up to 10 mg before bed, as it can reduce anxiety and promote sleep. This can be especially useful in the case of epileptics to decrease the severity of sleep disorders associated with the illness such as teeth grinding, nocturnal wandering and sleep apnoea but consideration for potential drug interactions has to be given with melatonin and certain anti-depressants.* ❞

There may be side effects of long-term use, and more research is needed to prove its safety for children. Sarah Newbury says, 'Treatment with melatonin should be initiated and supervised by a specialist, but may be continued by a GP under a shared-care arrangement. Treatment should be reviewed biannually.' She concludes, 'Short-term use of melatonin is well tolerated and useful where non-pharmacological interventions have been unsuccessful. Quality of family life can be significantly improved by improvements in quality and duration of sleep at night. Indeed, the improvement of daytime functioning could be considered the most important rationale for the use of sleep medication in children.'

Medication is definitely not the first route to explore if your child has sleep problems, and can cause unwanted daytime drowsiness. Doctors advise looking at eliminating daytime stimulants in food and drink first, and developing a good bedtime routine. If all possible other causes of disturbed sleep have first been eliminated, medication may then be considered.[17] Remember that many adult medications for sleep have not been approved for use in children. Sarah Newbury says:

> *In summary, the right treatment needs to be provided for the right patient, considering each case individually. Children with developmental delays, ADHD, autism and mood/anxiety disorders are more commonly prescribed sleep medications by clinicians or psychiatrists than GPs or paediatricians. Any change in dosage or dose times must be discussed with an appropriate healthcare professional first. Other changes to promote natural sleep should always be tried first and then used in conjunction with medication, for example, diet and nutritional counselling as well as behavioural therapy and stress management can help to relieve sleep problems.*

Do not buy herbal remedies for your child in the hope that they will improve sleep. Most remedies have not had the same level of testing as medicines, and do not have robust histories of safe use in children. Speak to a professional for advice first.

Sheila's son David has a diagnosis of autism. He has a range of issues associated with this, and has been using medication to help him sleep. Sheila says:

> *David doesn't sleep. He used to sleep more during the day as a baby. Now he head bangs for a short while to get himself to sleep which is distressing to listen to as a parent. We have a bedtime routine. He has been prescribed valergan forte and*

melatonin to help him sleep, so he has those between seven and half-past. On a good day it will take half an hour of head banging to get him off. If we have had a busy or stimulating day he can still be doing it three hours later. If you go into him he doesn't want you, he just wants to get to sleep and head banging is his way of doing it. If he wakes in the night he head bangs again which disturbs his brother. He may wake at two or at eleven and three. The meds do make a difference: we ran out of the valergan one night and it was much worse. "

Summary

In this chapter, you've learnt about how all sorts of daytime activities can affect your child's sleep. A sleep diary can help you work out what affects sleep, and you may want to complete a food diary too if you have concerns that this may play a role in sleep disturbances for your child. Write down what your child eats and drinks each day and see if it affects their sleep. Ask for help from a sleep specialist or a dietician if you are unsure. Simple strategies to implement include cutting out cola and other fizzy drinks or sugary snacks. Add in milky drinks, fruit and vegetables.

Exercise can help your child sleep too: pick high-intensity exercise a few hours before bed if your child has problems dropping off. If your child is a live wire, try out yoga classes for relaxation as well. Make sure your child gets plenty of exposure to morning light: try walking to school as that has the benefit of a little extra exercise plus light to help your child's body clock work well.

In the evening, remember to choose calming activities. Read Chapters 2 and 8 for more ideas for relaxation, and Chapters 1 and 5 for more on a good bedtime routine.

Finally, check if any of your child's medication may be keeping them awake. The information in this book is not exhaustive so talk to a pharmacist or your child's GP or paediatrician for specific advice. Changing the time your child takes their medication may help. For a small number of children medication can be used to help them sleep. Again, speak to a professional for advice on this before starting or stopping any medication.

Chapter 5
Bedtime Routine

In this chapter we explore the importance of establishing and maintaining a good bedtime routine in order to help with children's sleep issues, whether your child has a physical or developmental disability or other additional needs. You can also find out about what constitutes at good routine and get some ideas for activities to promote relaxation.

Establishing a happy and positive routine can be a wonderful way to end the day. The hour leading up to bedtime provides the perfect opportunity to share time with your child and to help them to relax. It is widely recognized that routine and structure helps children to feel safe and secure. For children with additional needs it also helps them to make sense of the time of day and to know what will happen next. A good bedtime routine is key to helping to support better sleep patterns. Don't panic if this sounds the complete opposite to your current run-up to bedtime. Read on to learn how small changes can make a big difference.

Dr Kairen Cullen is a chartered educational psychologist and tells us that all children can benefit greatly from routine. 'Children with additional needs, such as learning difficulties, have to cope with many challenges and this can increase anxiety, often expressed as frustration, anger and/or withdrawal. A consistent and appropriate bedtime routine will help them to feel more secure and calm, contribute to a good sleep and help them to cope better with their own specific challenges.'

As adults we often put routine into our day to help us to cope with challenges more effectively. If our routine is disrupted it can lead to us feeling unsettled. Think about a time when somebody sat in a chair that you usually sit in, or a time when you were running late and you weren't able to have your usual cup of coffee. How did these changes in your routine make you feel? Chances are that you didn't view them positively because even minor changes to routine can cause us to feel disorientated, frustrated or anxious.

Julie Sutton is an independent learning disability nurse and sleep practitioner trainer for the Handsel Project. She tells us:

    A child with a learning difficulty may need additional support to learn a consistent bedtime routine. It is essential to utilize the child's individual communication strategy to help them to calm down, self-soothe to sleep and understand the steps in a bedtime routine. For example, prepare a picture schedule showing bedtime activities in order which needs to be repeated every night, or design a Social Story about going to sleep to be read with the child every bedtime. It is important to consistently repeat the routine every night for a child with learning difficulties. Consistency and repetition help the child learn that bedtime is approaching and what is expected of them at night-time.

A good bedtime routine is about being consistent; the same thing should happen at the same time each day. A bedtime routine requires planning and in this chapter we explore how to design the perfect bedtime routine for your child using multi-sensory cues to support their understanding.

Circadian rhythm

In order to understand the importance of a bedtime routine it is necessary to explore the patterns of sleepiness that we all experience. We each have an internal body clock which regulates when we go to sleep. Some people may feel more alert in the morning and others in the evening; the internal body clock does have variations according to the individual.

We take our cues from the light which helps our bodies to produce a hormone called cortisol. When it becomes dark our bodies respond by producing another hormone called melatonin. It is melatonin that helps to make us feel sleepy and this is the reason that we suggest carrying out bedtime routines away from bright lighting; the aim is to promote melatonin production during the bedtime routine.

During adolescence there is a shift in the circadian rhythm and most teenagers experience a delayed sleep phase i.e. they want to go to sleep later at night but then find it difficult to get up the next morning. Research has shown that teenagers release melatonin later in the evening than other children and adults.

Although our days are twenty-four hours long it is interesting to note that our circadian rhythm actually runs on a longer cycle. Some researchers suggest this is just over twenty-four hours while others suggest it is closer to twenty-five hours. It is therefore important that we establish good bedtime routines in order to keep our bodies tuned in to the twenty-four hour clock. Children with a visual impairment may need additional cues in order to keep their bodies running in correlation with the twenty-four hour clock.

Claire says:

My son has severe visual impairment and nobody had explained to me the important role that light plays in our body clocks. Adam does not get these cues and therefore I have used a multi-sensory routine in order to build them in for him. The Children's Sleep Charity gave me support and I am pleased to say that his sleep is now much improved. Knowing this information has proved so important for us as a family and helped us support his sleep needs better.

Various bodily functions are connected with the sleep/wake cycle such as hormone secretion, blood pressure and the production of urine. It takes children's bodies some time to develop their own internal body clocks, though these should become established by the time a child is eighteen months old. Some research has suggested that children with autism spectrum disorders may not produce enough melatonin during the evenings, which can lead to sleep issues. There is also research that suggests that children with a diagnosis of ADHD may release melatonin later in the evening than other children: this will be explored in further detail in Chapter 9.

The right time?

Prior to thinking about what to include in a bedtime routine it is important to ensure that you are committed to carrying out the routine every night of the week. While routines are an excellent way of helping to support children's sleep problems they are also problematic in that they make demands on you as a parent.

Sarah explains:

❝ *My eldest son never had a routine and had terrible sleep issues. I just thought that he didn't need a great deal of sleep and decided to let him go to bed when he showed signs of being tired. After receiving support from a sleep practitioner I realized that he did need sleep and one of the major problems was that I'd never got him into a good routine at bedtime. My youngest son has therefore always had a good bedtime routine and has never had sleep issues. What I will say, however, is that maintaining the routine takes some hard work on our part. There is no nipping out for evening meals any longer or going to the shopping mall to pick up a last-minute gift. We have to make sure that we are home by 6 p.m. no matter what we are doing to start the routine. Our younger son is so routine-based that by 7 p.m. he is desperate to get in his bed and go to sleep. I hear lots of parents saying that they do a routine but it's a bit different every night and that makes me smile. A routine has to be the same each evening surely? Doing a routine can tie you down yet the bonus is that we have our evenings to ourselves.* ❞

This is an extremely important point that Sarah has made. A bedtime routine will take work on your part and your child may initially resist the new routine. You need to decide whether this is the right time for you as a family to implement a new routine and whether you have the resilience at this point in time to carry it out each evening.

Debbie has a daughter with Down's syndrome and explains how introducing a new bedtime routine seemed overwhelming:

❝ *When you are sleep deprived even the smallest of tasks seem enormous. I knew that I needed to implement a sleep routine for my daughter but I just couldn't actually face it. A practitioner supported me to identify a point in our lives when it would be easier to adopt a new routine, I opted for July ... we were only in January at the time! It took me six months to get myself into the right mindset to make the changes necessary, but I did it. By the time July came I was optimistic and ready to implement it. Looking back I'm glad that I did plan it and take my time, otherwise I think that I would have started it and given up. The good news is that having a routine made a significant difference to our lives and to my daughter's sleep habits. I'd advise other parents to do the same: plan the time when they are going to start to make the necessary changes.*

Beginning a new routine

You may wish to totally overhaul your child's bedtime routine or make small changes. Whatever you decide, you should plan the change and ensure that the new routine is motivating for your child. You are the expert on your child and will be best placed to decide whether they can cope with a completely new routine or whether it would be preferable to introduce small changes gradually.

It is important that when you do introduce a new routine that everybody involved in putting your child to bed is aware of the routine. It may be that you need to share the routine with grandparents, the respite centre or your child's other parent.

Jill tells us:

Sonny has learning difficulties and had horrendous sleep issues. Getting a bedtime routine in place was really helpful to get him to understand the difference between night and day. I have always carried out the routine while my husband sorted our other two children out. I recently went into hospital for a spell and realized in horror on my first night that I had never explained about Sonny's routine to my husband. I made a point of writing everything down that evening, down to the set phrases I tend to use so that the routine could be carried out in my absence. I think you just get so used to doing it yourself that sometimes you do forget to pass on the information and it really is very important information, particularly if you want to end the day well with some sleep! 〕〕

Emma Sweet is a sleep practitioner and works with families where children have disabilities. She says:

❝ *Sometimes it can be hard to make those changes but don't put too much pressure on yourself. If it is easier, just make one small change at a time. Rest assured that children do respond positively to bedtime routines, they like the structure and it helps them to feel safe and secure. Bedtime routines don't have to be elaborate and once you get a good bedtime routine it will be an enjoyable time to spend with your child.* 〕〕

Language and bedtime

Communication difficulties are common in children with additional needs. Children's language skills in general are significantly less developed than adults' and this impacts upon their understanding of instructions. Sometimes, therefore, it is challenging for parents to explain new routines to children.

Helen Gill is a specialist speech and language therapist and owns Time4talking, a company specializing in supporting the development of communication for children with additional needs. Helen tells us:

❝ *Children do not understand all the words that we say as parents. The fewer words that you use, the less filtering your child will need to do in order to understand. So, for example, a child will be far more likely to do what you ask if you say, 'It's bath time now, then pyjamas and story' rather than, 'Come on now, it's time to go upstairs for your bath and then we can get you into your pyjamas and then, because you've been really good today, we can take a look at that new book we got from the library.' Children are also highly distractible and their attention will naturally wander if instructions are too long-winded.* 〕〕

Sometimes it can be difficult to know exactly how much information to give our children at bedtime. Helen says:

" *A basic rule of thumb is to speak to your child with the same number of words that they use to communicate with you. If your child uses single words or signs to express themselves, then use single words or short phrases with them. If your child is currently non-verbal then keep your language to a minimum at all times and make sure you use visual cues to help your child understand. Objects of reference can be hugely helpful when giving instructions to a child who does not yet understand spoken language. If you consistently show them a bath sponge when you say 'bath' and put it on the bath, then over time your child will know that whenever they see the sponge that it is time to go for a bath.* "

We know that children learn this way because if you show a child their coat they will know that they are going outside; it's exactly the same principle.

Helen's top tips:
✓ Instructions should be short and simple
✓ You do not have to provide an explanation for what you are asking children to do, this can confuse them
✓ If you use objects of reference make sure that you use the same object for the same event
✓ Slow down your speech, children cannot process speech as quickly as adults deliver it
✓ Get your child's attention by using their name

Visual timetables

Time can be a confusing concept for children yet it is important to keep in mind throughout the bedtime routine. Helen says:

" *Children often learn best through visual means and therefore using pictures showing a sequence of events can be far more effective than saying a long list of events or instructions to a child. Visual timetables have a number of benefits when trying to help a child follow a sequence of events. Firstly, visual timetables can be as simple as you like. To start with they may just contain two tasks, for example, supper and bath time. As your child matures or becomes more used to using timetables the sequence can lengthen to include a number of tasks. Secondly, visual timetables remain in the here and now. A spoken word has gone the second it comes out of the speaker's mouth and there is nothing remaining for the child to focus on. A visual representation, such as a photograph, remains there and allows the child time to process and remember what they are doing next. Thirdly, visual timetables give the perception of control to the child. When implementing a bedtime routine the parent will be the one to decide the sequence and the events that will be included but the child has the chance to remove each of the pictures as they complete the task and post them into a 'bedtime box'. This means that the child is involved in the bedtime routine and has a sense of responsibility.* 🔳🔳

In order to use a visual timetable effectively your child needs to be able to select photographs from a choice of two. This means that when you ask them to give you or to look at a photograph they can identify the correct one around 80% of the time. If you are using photographs make sure that they are taken in good light and they are clear and uncluttered.

Some children prefer to work from the top down in sequence when using a timetable while other children prefer to work from left to right. If your child uses a visual timetable in school or pre-school it is a good idea to check with the practitioners to find out how the timetable is presented and whether photographs, symbols or objects of reference are used. It is important to replicate what is being used in other environments to support your child's understanding.

Making a visual timetable

You will need to use a piece of card as the base plate; getting this laminated will increase its durability. You will also need a selection of laminated symbols to use. You can use sticky backed Velcro to fix the cards onto the base plate.

Decide how many symbols you are going to have and break down the sequence of your bedtime routine. You may wish to include things like:

- ✓ Television time
- ✓ Tea
- ✓ Quiet time
- ✓ Supper
- ✓ Bath
- ✓ Toilet
- ✓ Pyjamas on
- ✓ Teeth cleaning
- ✓ Bedtime story
- ✓ Going to sleep

Your child should be encouraged to look at the timetable to identify what they are going to do next. If the next symbol is to clean teeth then your child should be encouraged to remove this from the chart and to take it with them to the sink. You may wish to have a copy of the same symbol by the sink for your child to match so that they know that they have followed the timetable accurately. Alternatively you may wish to make a post box for your child to put the symbols into once they have carried out the activity.

Helen advises that sometimes it is useful to use sand timers during the bedtime routine.

" Visual timers can be useful to let your child know how long they can remain on a task particularly if it is something they like and are unlikely to be willing to come away from. Also these can be useful to motivate children to do tasks that they have little interest in so that they realize that they don't have to stay there forever! "

Dave used a sand timer for his daughter who is eight years old and has autism and challenging behaviour.

❝ *Sienna loves her television, in fact so much so that she has three televisions all on different channels playing at once. I realized that this was problematic in the run-up to bedtime and every night there would be a battle to get her to turn them off. It was suggested that I use a sand timer so that she gets a warning that television time is coming to an end. I'm not saying that it was easy initially but she did learn the rule fairly quickly and now when the sand runs out she will usually turn off the televisions in a calm manner.* ❞

Screens and bedtime

Any kind of screen activity such as using a computer, television or mobile phone is highly stimulating and best avoided in the lead-up to bedtime. Dr Kairen Cullen says:

❝ *Video games and television programmes can stimulate the child in such a way that they can find it hard to wind down and relax enough to sleep. Inappropriate viewing material can even contribute to disturbed sleep and nightmares. One of the main functions of sleep is that of processing and accommodating an individual's emotional experiences. If sleep or quality of sleep is reduced by excessive, unsupervised computer-game playing and television viewing, especially when it is too close to bedtime, the harmful effects are increased yet further.* ❞

Research has consistently shown a link between children engaging in screen activities prior to bed and them getting less sleep. The white light from screens is also noted to interfere with melatonin production and therefore hinder nodding off.

Many parents use the television as part of the bedtime routine. If your child has a sleep problem it is recommended that they do not have access to screens in the hour leading up to bedtime.

Tips for limiting screen time

So how do you limit screens? Consider the following:

✓ Remove all computers, televisions and mobile phones from the bedroom.

✓ Put screen time into the early part of the routine so that your child still gets to engage in the activity

✓ Give your child verbal warnings that the screen time is going to end soon

✓ Use a visual cue if needs be, such as a clock or sand timer

✓ Reward your child for positively ending the sessions

✓ Make sure that you have something interesting to offer them to do as an alternative

John's son has autism and he was extremely worried about turning off the television in the evening.

" *I was very reluctant to follow this advice as I knew that Tom would kick off if the television was being turned off. I did however give it a go and was really surprised at the results. Yes, Tom didn't like the fact that his viewing time was being limited but by day three I noticed that he was much calmer in himself and he started to settle more quickly at bedtime.* "

Setting the scene

It is important that during the lead-up to bedtime all televisions are switched off in the house and that a calm, relaxing environment is created. Dimming the lights can be useful in aiding the production of melatonin and encouraging your child to learn that the end of the day is fast approaching.

Many children respond positively to the use of music within a bedtime routine. Music has been found to have a profound effect on the health and well-being of children. Several studies have shown that children have presented with increased activity levels when they have listened to fast music.[18] Relaxing music on the other hand has been found to improve behaviour.[19] Background music has been shown to have an impact on lowering stress levels; for example, some research has shown that listening to music prior to surgery can reduce anxiety in day surgery patients.

Emma Sweet tells us:

  Music can be particularly useful when incorporated into a good bedtime routine. For children who can't tell the time it can give them an auditory signal that bedtime is approaching. When used alongside a good bedtime routine music has been found to have an extremely positive impact on mood, behaviour and sleep, not only of the child but also of the parent. Bedtime is stressful in many households; music can help to create a more positive and relaxing environment. Music can also help to mask the sound of other noises in the environment such as children playing outside or the television on in the next room!

The Children's Sleep Charity offers a CD using the latest in scientific research to promote relaxation at bedtime. *Night and Day the Easy Way* has been developed in order to help children to unwind during the bedtime routine. Composer Catherine Rannus from Belightful Music has produced the two tracks for the charity, one for the morning and one for the evening. Catherine tells us:

  Research has shown that music can have a positive effect on the mind and help to calm or energize. Using the latest scientific research I created two contrasting pieces of music for children, one for bedtime to help them to relax and one for the morning to energize them ready for the day ahead. By experimenting with the number of beats per minute in the music and altering the pitch a unique listening experience has been created to support a better night's sleep.

Nigel Allen is a special-needs teacher and explains how his pupils often respond positively to music:

  I think music can be extremely powerful and find that my pupils often respond very well to it. I use it to give them some understanding of the time of day. Time can be a very confusing concept for children with additional needs. I use a set piece each morning so that when they enter the classroom they have an idea of what will be happening next. I also use a set piece at the end of the day. I find that it helps to develop a sense of time and routine so I can see that use of music within the bedtime routine would be helpful for some families. 〞

If you do use music within the bedtime routine ensure that you turn it off before your child goes to sleep. If they fall asleep listening to music then they are likely to wake up once they have been through a sleep cycle if it has ceased. The aim is to keep conditions throughout the night consistent to minimize any night wakings.

Some children also respond positively to the use of fragrances within the bedtime routine in order to again give them a sense of time. Using a certain smell at a set time can indicate that bedtime is approaching and may help to prepare them for the bedtime routine.

Pre-bedtime activities

So with the screens switched off it is time to engage your child in some relaxing activities prior to bed. It may be that initially you can only engage in a few minutes of these activities and that you build up the length of time spent on them gradually each day. The activities that you choose should be motivating and interesting for your child otherwise they will not want to take part in them. First of all, consider what your child is interested in. It may be a cartoon character, a sport or a more specialist interest. Think creatively to see if you can tie in their interests with appropriate calming activities. We give you some examples below.

First of all make sure that you have a nice relaxing space to encourage your child to wind down in. Offer them a selection of activities to choose from if appropriate. This period of time should be calming so physical activities should be avoided.

Possible activities

Hand–eye co-ordination activities are excellent for promoting relaxation. Think of all the adults you know who engage in pursuits such as sewing or knitting! Below are examples of suitable activities that you may consider:

✓ Threading
✓ Jigsaws
✓ Building bricks
✓ Dough
✓ Colouring in
✓ Dressing a doll
✓ Sewing

For children with fine motor-skill difficulties finger rhymes can be helpful as can hand massage. Sensory stories are also a lovely way of winding down and children can be encouraged to feel the different textures throughout the books.

You will find more information about relaxing activities in Chapter 8 of this book.

Bathing within the routine

Do you like a bath before you go to sleep? For many children a bath can help them wind down and relax. It provides a useful transition time from the day's activities to bedtime too.

Having a bath at bedtime can excite or frighten children. Hayley says:

❝ *Josh used to scream the house down every night when I bathed him. I carried on doing it because I just thought that it was the right thing to do! It turned out that he was actually terrified of the water so far from it being a relaxing activity it was a traumatic one. It was the health visitor who suggested that I move it out of the bedtime routine. It was such a simple change to make but made a lot of difference. I can't believe looking back I carried on doing it to be honest but you just try to do the best for your child and I thought I was doing the right thing at the time.* ❞

If your child becomes stressed by bath time then it is a good idea to move it away from the bedtime routine if at all possible. Some children find bath time over-stimulating and will get extremely excited in the bath; again, if this is the case, you may wish to consider moving it to another time slot. Others find ending bath time too upsetting, again if it causes your child to get upset when bath time is over you could move the time slot.

For many children, however, bath time can provide a wonderful way to relax during the bedtime routine. Ideally you should aim to bathe your child around half an hour before they fall asleep. The bath will increase their body temperature and this will then slowly decrease as they get ready for bed. It is this decrease in body temperature that leads them to feel sleepy. A warm bath can also help to accelerate the release of melatonin. There are many bath products on the market for children that claim to help to promote sleep.

Bedtime stories

Reading your child a bedtime story can be a lovely way to end the day, as long as your child enjoys this time. It is important that you set a time limit on how long you are going to read the story for. Some stories can over-excite or stimulate children and are best avoided in the bedtime routine.

Jenna says, 'My son loves Thomas the Tank Engine. I have to avoid telling Thomas stories at all costs in the run-up to bedtime as he just gets over-excited and starts to act them out in detail.'

There are many audio books and relaxation CDs on the market that may prove useful. It is important to ensure that the story finishes while your child is awake so that they learn to fall asleep independently. If they fall asleep with you reading them a story they are likely to wake up later in the evening because conditions have changed.

Saying goodnight

Giving hugs and kisses at bedtime is wonderful although some children may try to extend this period. Using a set phrase to end the session can be extremely useful such as 'It's time to sleep' or 'It's night-time, go to sleep now'. This will signal to your child that you are about to leave and that you are not going to engage in further conversation.

Changes to routine

There will undoubtedly be periods of time where your bedtime routine cannot be followed. Christmas is an example of when most routines go out of the window, as are family holidays. Also if your child is ill you may find it more difficult to stick to a routine. If you do set up a routine and it goes off track, don't worry about it; simply consider why this has happened and then adjust the routine to meet the new circumstances.

As children develop you may need to adjust the routine. For example, your child may need to go to bed later as they get older and you may need to tweak the activities that you offer in order for them to remain interesting.

The clocks changing can also cause difficulties with children's sleep routines. In the spring we lose an hour's sleep as the clocks move forwards and in the winter we gain an hour's sleep. For some children it is helpful if you plan for this change by gradually changing the time that they go to bed over a period of a few weeks. So for example when we lose an hour's worth of sleep in the springtime you should start putting your child to bed fifteen minutes earlier each week in the month leading up to the change. By the time the clocks change your child's body clock will be fully synchronized. Making these small changes can be extremely helpful. Then you simply reverse the process in the wintertime and put your child to bed fifteen minutes later.

It may be tempting to ditch the bedtime routine at the weekend or to try to keep your child up later so that you get a lie-in. Unfortunately this will not help with their sleep issues. A bedtime routine needs to be carried out consistently and you should try not to deviate from your child's bedtime if at all possible. It is highly likely that even if you do put them to bed later they will still get up at the same time in the morning!

The getting-up routine

While most parents are very aware of what time their children should be in bed, many are unclear about what time they should be getting up. It is very important that you consider what is a reasonable time to start the day and that you wake your child at this set time each day if they are not already awake. This will help to strengthen their internal body clock and help them to develop better sleep habits. It will also help you to determine whether you are dealing with a night-time waking or you are actually starting the day. It is important to be realistic about getting-up time. It is not unreasonable for children to wake from 6.30 a.m. onwards if they have had a good night's sleep.

Cara has a son with learning difficulties and tells us:

" Getting my son up at a set time each day was actually key in helping with his sleep problems. I was so worn out that I just let him stay in bed if he wasn't awake; this clearly impacted on his night-time sleep. Getting him up was difficult for us both but I did notice a difference quite quickly and he started to go to bed earlier as a result. "

When you wake your child make sure that you let light into the room. Put the lights on if it is wintertime and draw back the curtains.

Summary

A good bedtime routine is an important way of supporting better sleeping habits. Carrying out a bedtime routine should be a pleasant experience for both you and your child. The key to developing a good routine is consistency and using activities that your child enjoys so that they are keen to engage.

It is important that the same routine is carried out at the same time every night. Children with additional needs enjoy routine as it makes them feel safe and secure. Our aim at bedtime is to promote relaxation and feelings of security. In Chapter 10 we will provide you with a template to plan your own bedtime routine.

Chapter 6
Sleep and the Bedroom Environment

If you're reading this book, it is likely that your child struggles to sleep. It is vital to read the first few chapters so you can discover behavioural techniques to help improve your child's sleep, but the bedroom environment can play an important role too. All too often we forget about the importance of creating the right setting for your child to fall asleep in. Read this chapter to find out more about how you can make your child's bedroom a relaxing retreat from the outside world that will enhance their sleep. You will also find out more about environmental factors such as light and noise that may be preventing your child from sleeping.

In the second half of the chapter, we move beyond the regular bedroom environment and look at specialist equipment that will help children with additional needs, as well as getting funding towards this sort of equipment.

Tim is ten and has a combination of additional needs. His mum describes his bedroom:

" Tim has the biggest bedroom in the house. Cream and blue, blue blackout blind and curtains, blue carpet. There is no TV but he does have a computer which he uses to watch films or Lego videos amongst other things. Lots and lots of Lego – we have now drawn out an area for Lego and marked it with silver tape on the floor – the idea is the Lego should stay in that segment.... It is a work in progress! Tim has a number of things in his room to help him chill out and wind down. He has a gym ball and theraband for OT exercises. Tim also uses his gym ball instead of a chair at his desk. We had a dimmer switch fitted to the main light. I would love to incorporate some other interesting objects which would help Tim 'reset'

his senses: some that give out light e.g. fibre optic things, rope lights etc., some which help with the auditory side – speakers and music etc., and some which envelop him, generating feelings of security e.g. a hammock chair or big beanbag – we are currently saving up! Other things: there is a big map of the world on his wall, all of his books are in there, and obviously his clothes. 〞

What makes a relaxing bedroom?

Is your child's bedroom a relaxing place, or is it full of bright colours or cluttered with toys or noisy electronic games? Take a moment to think how you might feel if you had to sleep in your child's room. Would you complain about the uncomfortable bed? The way the light shines in from dawn? Or the noise of the early morning delivery lorry?

Then think about what might make a relaxing bedroom. Tear out pictures from catalogues and magazines or browse photo sites like Pinterest for ideas. Look at the rooms you have picked out. What sort of colours seem relaxing? What sort of décor? Think about rooms where you have had a great night's sleep. Were they quiet? Dark? What about when your child has actually slept well? The more you can identify helpful factors, the better night's sleep that can be achieved. Read on for more inspiration.

Assessing your child's bedroom and making changes

What's in the room?

Take a good look at your child's bedroom. Many children find their bedrooms over-stimulating and benefit from sleeping in a low arousal environment. When you put them to bed at night do they see everything that they have been playing with? This can remind them that staying awake is more fun than going to sleep. This will affect different children to different degrees but spending five minutes putting toys in boxes and closing cupboard doors can signal the end of playtime and create a calmer environment. This will encourage your child to drop off with less fuss. If you have a lot of toys, buy some storage boxes if you need to, and consider putting some toys elsewhere in the house. You could donate some toys to charity or use loft or garage space to pack away toys that are less popular and rotate which boxes you bring out. Set aside a day to declutter your child's bedroom: by doing so you can make space to add in items to aid relaxation, such as family photos. Read on for more ideas.

Does your child watch TV in their room?

It can be easy to allow your child to have a television in their bedroom, and sometimes a TV programme can become part of your child's bedtime routine. But watching television or playing computer games can stimulate the brain. The increased light levels from electronic devices has an impact on hormone production and interferes with signals to our bodies to switch off for the night. This can stop your child from winding down, and ultimately prevent them from sleeping.

Consider whether your child really needs a TV or computer in their bedroom. It may be better to take it out and to watch it in another room. If this wouldn't work for your child, another option is to have a strict deadline for the TV to go off, and use a blanket or towel to cover it up to remind your child that TV time is over. A timer switch can prevent your child switching it on again.

Bedroom temperature

How hot is your child's room? Make sure that the temperature in the bedroom is comfortable. Consider whether the room gets hot or cold at night. Use a thermometer and check the temperature when you go to bed and when your child wakes. A min-max thermometer will measure the minimum and maximum temperature that the room reaches, so you can check it in the morning. Ideally the bedroom should be slightly cooler than ambient daytime temperature; around 65°F or 18°C. If the room is getting very cold, is your child waking because they are cold? Similarly, if your child has a tendency to overheat, can they remove some of their covers themselves? Some children have particular difficulties regulating their own temperature: this may be the case if your child has a metabolic disorder, is fighting off an infection or has difficulty sweating. Ask yourself whether this is affecting your child. An overweight child may be inclined to feel hot, while an underweight one may struggle to stay warm enough. Some medications can affect the way your child feels the cold too.

Nell says:

> ❝ *The boys' room is at the back of the house, which faces north. It is definitely colder than the rest of the house, and when we first moved in I worried that they would get cold. We have a thermostat that controls the heating, and it's moveable, so I solved my worries by moving the thermostat to their bedroom. Everyone else seems fine: my south-facing bedroom is warmer, but I can easily adjust the radiator, and I know that the boys' room temperature will be fairly constant.* ❞

Your child's body will naturally respond to a lowering body temperature as they fall asleep. This is why a hot bath before bed, which raises the body temperature, can help your child drop off. If your child is too hot and cannot regulate their temperature, either by sweating or by removing layers of clothing or bedding, this can hinder the process of getting to sleep. Give your child loose, light cotton nightwear and use a number of layers of thin bedding rather than one thick layer. Consider purchasing a fan or air-conditioning unit.

Memory foam mattresses respond to body temperature. Higher-density memory foam softens in reaction to body heat, allowing it to mould to a warm body. Some people find that they overheat more when using a memory foam mattress. If your child wakes when they are cold, they may be kicking off the covers or stripping out of their sleepwear. Look into the range of sleep suits and sleeping bags which are now available in a range of sizes. Duvets work by trapping in warm air to keep the body heated. If your child is prone to overheating they may be better with more thinner layers of bedding rather than a duvet. See the specialist equipment section later in this chapter for more information about bedding options.

There are lots more ways to adjust your child's room temperature from the very simple to those which will require a tradesman. If the room gets hot, leave the window slightly open so that air can circulate.

Make sure that it will only open an inch or so, and use window clips to restrict your child from opening it all the way. If you have old radiators they may not have individual thermostats. Adding in radiator thermostats will help you control the heat in each bedroom individually, which would help in Nell's situation (left).

If you are concerned that heating is making your child's bedroom dry you could buy a humidifier. Plants in the room can also help to produce oxygen and can bring moisture into dry environments. Some children will find this helpful, particularly if they take medication that can lead to a dry mouth.

From light to dark

As mentioned above in relation to televisions and other electronic devices, the body takes the onset of darkness as a sign to produce melatonin. In humans, melatonin comes from the pineal gland, which is in the centre of the brain. Melatonin sends a chemical signal to regulate the sleep–wake cycle, causing drowsiness and lowering the body temperature too (see page 13). Babies only develop regular melatonin levels in about the third month after birth. As we age, we produce less melatonin: in teenagers it is thought that the time at which melatonin is produced shifts, leading to later sleep and wake times.

Light is fundamental to the cycle of melatonin production. As it hits the back of the eye it inhibits melatonin production by the pineal gland, until the onset of darkness begins again. You can assist your child to feel sleepy by drawing the curtains, particularly on summer nights when it is light for longer. It is also important to make sure that your child gets daylight in the morning, which will help them wake and feel tired at an appropriate time later on in the day.

Look at your child's bedroom at different times of day. Does it get early morning light, which might cause your child to wake early, or is it sunny in the evening, hampering their efforts to go to sleep? A dark bedroom can increase the amount of melatonin that your child's body creates which makes them feel drowsy.

Practically, there are a number of ways to make your child's bedroom darker. Assess the curtains that you use – do they block out the light? While pretty light-coloured curtains may fit with the décor, you can boost their effectiveness with blackout blinds to make sure that the early morning light does not creep in and cause your child to wake up, particularly during the summer months. Experiment with a blanket or thick towel on top of the curtains and see if this encourages your child to sleep in a little longer.

There are many sorts of blackout blinds from ones that need permanent fixing to portable ones suitable for holidays and ones you can cut to fit awkward-shaped windows. You can find blinds that attach with Velcro which you stick to the window frame, as well as those that use suckers to attach to any window. The Velcro attachments have the advantage of minimizing gaps where light can enter round the side of the blind, but of course the Velcro needs to be stuck to the frame on a semi-permanent basis. If you love the curtains you have already you can add in blackout-quality linings which come in black, cream or white. Blackout fabric roller blinds are also available in a range of colours and patterns. You can cut this sort of blind to fit your window: you may need a small hacksaw if the inner tube has to be adjusted. Use with safety hooks to keep the sidewinder cord out of the reach of children. Look at www.easyblindsonline.co.uk for mail order, ideas and inspiration. There are also blinds which stick to windows using statically charged polypropylene film. The blind sheets come in a roll, and can be torn off and cut to fit. They last around six to eight weeks if in daily use and have to be put up at night then removed in the morning. See www.magicblackoutblind.co.uk for more information. In general, blackout blinds can cost between £14 and £50, depending on the size and type of blind.

Don't forget: many items of electrical equipment have LED lights to indicate if they are charging or on standby. These lights can prevent your child's bedroom from getting fully dark, and some may flash which is particularly disturbing. Remove them, switch them off at the mains or cover them if safe to do so. This also applies to the light from digital clocks which can be intrusive. You can simply stand a card in front of the clock to see if that produces fuller darkness.

If you are considering what else you can do to help your child wind down at night, or if you have a child who struggles to relax in total darkness, consider changing the light bulbs for a lower wattage, or swapping to a dimmer switch. A dimmer switch can allow you to control the amount of light used at different times of the day. You may decrease the light level as your child changes for bed, then take it down a little further as they lie in bed, before switching it off altogether when it is time to go to sleep.

Some families need to change or give feeds during the night. Putting on a bright light can wake both you and your child. Try using a glowing light in a different colour to white. A red, blue or orange light bulb, for example, can give enough light to see but not enough to wake your child fully.

Remember that some children may not cope with a fully darkened room. This may be a particular issue for children with visual or hearing impairment.

Colours for sleep

What colour is your child's bedroom? The colour of the bedroom can have an impact on the quality of your child's sleep. Think about the typical colours used in many of your child's toys. Bright colours tend to dominate a child's world, and that's great when it's playtime. But if you have ever eaten in a fast-food restaurant, surrounded by red, yellow and orange, and wondered why the children gobble their food and then want to run around, just look at the walls. Bright colours tend to be less restful. Fast-food chains use bright colours to speed up people so they eat and leave rapidly, and the restaurant can serve more diners. So appreciate that if your child's bedroom is full of bright colours they may well find it harder to wind down.

If your child's bedroom is full of bright toys, we have already talked about putting them into boxes for the night. You could even use a plain sheet to cover stimulating, bright and exciting toys up.

But what about the walls and curtains? Plain white walls reflect the maximum amount of light. You could think about toning down bright colours: one example of this is to repaint a bright pink girly bedroom in pale pink and lilac tones. You'll find a complete change in the atmosphere. And soft colours can work well for boys – choose pastel blues and greens for a calming room, or pale green and beige for one with a nature theme that will work for both genders. Consider this when you are next redecorating.

Hot colours, are also often stimulating colours	Cool colours, tend also to be calming colours
Bright pink Red Orange Yellow	Pale pink Purples and lilacs Dark and pale blues Green Grey White Beige

Noise

Is your child's room quiet or noisy? Think about its location. Does your child hear everyone walking past as they go to the bathroom? Do they get noise from the main road? Can they hear an older sibling playing music in their bedroom, or the TV from downstairs? Any of these noises can make it harder for your child to drop off, or may cause waking in the night. Noise can be a particular issue for children with sensory sensitivity: noises that you easily ignore may bother them, even if it is something as quiet as the hum of a computer monitor on standby or the refrigerator downstairs.

Not every child is affected by this issue: some might find it hard to get to sleep without the comforting noise of the family around them, but do experiment. A night spent sleeping in your child's room may show you that the traffic starts up just around the same time they always wake you!

There are some quick fixes to help create a quiet environment for sleep, and some that require a little more investment or inconvenience. Start by sitting and listening while your child is dropping off to sleep. Sit just outside their room and note down what you can hear. What is making a noise in their room? Is there a ticking clock? Does your child like this, or would they be happier without its sound? Could you cut some noise by simply closing the door to the kitchen, so they cannot hear the washing machine or refrigerator? Closing the door to the lounge will keep out noise from adults who are still awake, chatting or watching television.

Ask older siblings to keep the noise down, particularly around the hour that your child is dropping off. You could suggest that they go downstairs if your house is on two floors, just for the time that your younger child is doing their bedtime routine and dropping off to sleep. Offer a new pair of headphones as an incentive to keep the evening as quiet time.

If you have lots of noise coming through a wall, whether it joins a neighbouring house, or just a noisy older child's bedroom, consider moving the furniture. Add shelves and wardrobes to the wall where noise seeps through. Wardrobes full of clothes will provide the most insulation. You could try temporary measures first then consider getting fitted wardrobes, and even adding in a layer of insulation between the back of the wardrobe and the wall. Remember to allow space for air to circulate.

Fabric absorbs sound, while hard surfaces reflect it, so changing the décor in your child's bedroom will change the noise levels. If you have hard floors and blinds, carpet and curtains will absorb sound more effectively. A thicker carpet will be more effective than a thin mat. Add in cushions too, if you want.

If your child's room is at the noisier side of the house, what would happen if you switched the rooms where people slept? Moving your child's bedroom can seem disruptive but may have long-term benefits.

If your child has problems dropping off to sleep, they may enjoy listening to their own choice of relaxing music. Look at relaxation CDs and story CDs and see if this helps your child.

Rebecca says, 'Music helps my 7-year-old son who has ADHD. We have tried all sorts to help Joe settle and music was the one thing that helped. He has an iPod and puts his headphones on. He finds listening to his favourite artists helps him. He's a fan of Depeche Mode and Pet Shop Boys believe it or not!'

You may want to try out a white-noise machine. This creates a low hum, like a hoover, and can block out other noises. You can find white-noise machines from between £20 and £60. Some are designed specifically for children: either as simple sound-producing boxes or the Prince Lionheart Slumber Bear that produces womb sounds, lullabies, ocean waves and white noise. A cheaper alternative is to buy a

CD or download a white-noise track for your own player. And a fan in the bedroom may have similar effects. If your child falls to sleep with noise they may need it to be consistent throughout the night to avoid them waking up after a sleep cycle.

If you have single-layer glass windows, double glazing will definitely reduce the noise in your house. This is obviously a big investment so you will want to try other things first. Alternatively, if you have been considering double glazing for some time, this may be the spur you need to do it.

Bedding and comfort at night

Is your child comfortable in bed at night? If you have ever slept in an uncomfortable bed, you'll know how this can affect your sleep. Similarly, if you have been in pain you'll understand it can loom much larger at night-time. There are many elements to getting comfortable at night and we will look at these in this section.

Emotionally, what does your child need to be relaxed? A good bedtime routine will help them wind down, and a cuddle and kiss will leave them feeling emotionally reassured. Younger children can gain emotional reassurance from a favourite soft toy too.

On the other hand, arguments at bedtime can leave your child emotionally on edge. This is also the case if they end up thinking about difficult situations. Try to address any issues arising from school on the way home so they have time to work through any problems with work or friends. This is better than it all coming up at bedtime.

Physically speaking, the bed is key to a good night's sleep. Some children seem happy to sleep with a range of books and toys in bed with them, but a comfortable bed can make a big difference.

Look at your child's mattress. Is it comfortable when you try it? When was the last time you turned it? Turning a mattress every week or month will ensure it wears better and lasts longer as well as keeping it comfortable for longer.

Check the instructions on the mattress. Because children grow rapidly, you may need to replace their mattress more frequently. A lightweight foam mattress which was fine for a small toddler may not provide the best support for a hefty teenager. A pocket-sprung mattress is the most costly option, but provides more support and is longer lasting for an older and larger child or teen. The mattresses included with some children's beds may not be robust and support-ive. When did you last replace your child's mattress? Generally, it is advised that you replace a mattress every seven to ten years. Take your child with you to choose a mattress if you can: you may be sur-prised by their views on which one is more comfortable. See if they can roll over comfortably too. Choose a washable waterproof mat-tress cover at the same time as you choose the new mattress to make sure that it is protected from day one.

Roberta's daughter frequently got out of bed during the night and went to sleep on the floor. Roberta was extremely concerned about this and repeatedly put her daughter back into bed, only for her to wake and go back to sleep on the floor.

I never really considered why she was getting up in the night until I discussed this with a sleep practitioner. My daughter always slept well on the floor but it just didn't seem right to leave her there. I was asked about her sensory needs and it soon became apparent that she sleeps well at her dad's house where the mattress is firm. I had been and bought a very soft mattress because that's what I prefer. What I now realize is that she has a preference for a firm mattress and she was trying to communicate this to me by moving during the night to the floor! I've since changed the mattress to a firmer one and she has stopped the midnight wanderings.

Another area that affects comfort but is easy to neglect is your child's pillow. Children benefit from thinner pillows than adults, and chil-dren who sleep on their backs are likely to need a thinner pillow than those who sleep on their side. You may want to get machine-washable pillows, particularly if your child still dribbles at night. Pillow covers are also available and can save you from washing the pillow so often.

Look at your child's duvet. What tog is it? If you live in a house where the temperature drops significantly on winter nights you may want a thicker duvet for this time of the year. All duvets are given a warmth rating which is measured in togs. The higher the tog the warmer the duvet. If you live in a modern, well-insulated house where the temperature rarely drops much at night, or your child is naturally warm, they may prefer a thinner duvet. There are also combination duvets that can be used as single spring- or summer-weight duvets or combined to make a thicker winter-weight duvet. A duvet's warmth comes from the way it retains warm air in tiny pockets within the filling. Shaking up the duvet every day will ensure that it remains warm. Breathable duvets are another option; these are made of more natural fabrics. See www.welovesleep.co.uk for breathable duvets.

If you suspect your child is waking due to pain, talk to their specialist. Pain-relieving medication can be delivered in slow-release forms which are better suited for overnight and can prevent your child waking in discomfort. If you have to wake your child to give them medication, ask the pharmacist if there is an alternative: you may be able to tweak the times at which you give the medication, or there may be slow-release options.

See the section on specialist equipment (right) for more ideas on getting your child comfortable at night.

Scent to help sleep

Did you know we still go on smelling while we sleep? It makes sense that a bad smell might put you off going to sleep, but certain scents may contribute to a good night's sleep. It has been shown that breathing scents like rosemary and lavender has an effect on the brain's activity. If you are desperate to get your child to drop off, think about ways that scent can add to a calm atmosphere. For children who are sensitive to scent, it can act as a strong signal that it is time to wind down and go to sleep.

A pilot study showed that lavender may improve insomnia.[20] Another study on children with autism at a residential school did not show a benefit from aromatherapy massage with lavender oil, but the authors state that more research is needed. [21]

Aromatherapy uses essential oils to promote physical and emotional well-being. There are a number of ways to explore whether scent will help your child to sleep. Mohdoh makes mouldable dough infused with oils thought to contribute to sleep. You can get lavender as a linen spray for sheets. Use oils like roman chamomile or lavender oil in the bath, diluted in massage oil, or put a couple of drops of oil onto a handkerchief and place it inside your child's pillowcase. Aromatherapy oils can be bought in health stores. Always read the instructions carefully before using them. Do not use undiluted oils directly on your child's skin. Visit an aromatherapist for further advice. The General Regulatory Council For Complementary Therapies (GRCCT) or the Complementary and Natural Healthcare Council (CNHC) can help you find a qualified practitioner. Read more about aromatherapy and other therapies to help your child relax in Chapter 8.

Specialist equipment

Sensory bedroom lighting

If your child has sensory sensitivity, sensory-processing disorder or one of the many conditions associated with this, you may have taken them to use a sensory room. A sensory room is a place where children and adults with special needs can explore and develop their senses and skills. It can provide an oasis of calm for your child. While setting up a sensory room can be expensive, there are some parts of the sensory room experience that can translate to your child's bedroom and help make it a place that they can wind down. A bubble or lava lamp, a projector, or a mobile can act as a sign to your child that it is wind-down time or give them something to watch while they are going to sleep. A fibre optic light can also fascinate some children. These lights cost in the region of £10–£30. Make sure that lights are out of reach of your child, and switch them off before they drop off to sleep, unless you plan to keep the lights on all night.

Weighted blankets for children with sensory impairment

Some children with sensory-processing and motor-planning issues find that weighted blankets help them self-calm. These can be a useful resource for children with ADHD/ADD, Asperger's syndrome, autism or ASD, but can also help children with conditions such as cerebral palsy, Down's syndrome or Rett syndrome with a sensory-processing element. Children can find a weighted blanket comforting as it helps their body relax and indicates to the autonomic nervous system to slow down. The deep pressure can have a calming effect and promote a sense of well-being which encourages relaxation and better sleep. Some children will have an improved sense of body position. Children who benefit from a weighted blanket at night may also find a weighted lap pad helps them calm down during the day, and there are weighted jackets and belts available if this strategy is successful for your child.

Talk to your child's therapist before trying a weighted blanket for guidance on safe and appropriate use. The size and weight of the blanket will depend on your child's size and weight. Blankets range in weight from 2 lb to 25 lb: the blanket of choice for a small child would be very different to one that would suit a large, tall teenager. Make sure that your child is able to remove their own blanket should they need to. A blanket should never cover the child's head. Different blankets use different systems to provide weight, from plastic balls sewn into fabric pouches to gel weights.

There are a range of blankets available, costing from £50 to several hundred pounds for custom designs. Some blankets have pockets to allow distribution of the weights to suit your child, while in others the weights are sewn in. Check on the availability of spare weights and covers. Look at www.kingkraft.co.uk for a good range of blankets. See the section below on funding for equipment if your child needs a blanket that cannot be prescribed by their therapist on the NHS. You may want to opt for a blanket that is CE marked and registered with the MHRA (Medical and Healthcare Regulatory Agency) as a medical device. This type of blanket would be VAT exempt, while you may still pay VAT on blankets that are not registered as medical devices. Do not use a weighted blanket without input from an occupational therapist.

Quick-change night-time bedding

Wet bedding and clothes can be a key cause of broken nights for some families. If your child is prone to leaks at night, look for draw sheets that can be placed over the regular sheets and changed quickly and easily, without the need for the whole bed to be changed. Nell says:

I've used Brollysheets. They tuck in either side and are made of multiple layers of fabric with a soft cotton top. I like them because they are easier to change and wash than a full set of sheets. "

Coverdry fleece wraps can be used at night as well as on a chair in the daytime. Waterproof sheets, duvets and pillow protectors are also a good investment, and upgrade to wipe-clean pillows and duvets if your child is prone to leaks at night.

Waterproof mattress covers are widely available online and locally from just a few pounds, but look at Fledglings (see page 114) and search on Amazon for more specific products designed for children with additional needs. There are also disposable bed mats/draw sheets available if you prefer, and Fledglings sell wipe-clean mattresses.

Beyond equipment to make dealing with leaks easier, you may want to look for help to improve your child's night-time continence. If your child is incontinent and you are not getting help, ask your GP for referral to your local continence service. You may also be able to self-refer. Each area will have their own guidelines on the prescription of continence products on the NHS, but you will get some help and advice. There is a useful factsheet about suppliers of continence products from Promocon at www.promocon.co.uk and www.disabledliving.co.uk.

ERIC works to improve the quality of life of children, young people and their families in the UK who suffer from the conse-quences of childhood incontinence, and to help them manage or overcome these problems. See www.eric.org.uk for further details. The charity has a website full of advice and offers a range of products to help in its shop, from bedding protection and alarms to protectors for when your child is away for the night. The range also includes sleep suits and books to help children with the issues raised by incon-tinence and bed-wetting.

Specialist sleep wear for children who remove clothing during the night

One of the causes of night waking may be that your child has removed their clothing, and then wakes up cold later on. If they still wear nappies at night this can cause even more problems. Look for all-in-one sleepwear to make this less likely. Many parents are frustrated when their child outgrows all-in-ones made for babies and toddlers. There are sleep suits available in larger sizes, albeit at a higher cost. You'll find lots of useful clothing including unitards, popper vests and all-in-one sleep suits in the Fledglings catalogue, which also offers a made-to-measure service. Fledglings is a national charity which aims to improve the lives of disabled children, and the products they sell are not priced for profit. Find out more about the charity and its services at www.fledglings.org.uk or read the catalogue www.fledglings.org.uk/docs/pdf/brochure.pdf.

If you need larger size all-in-one pyjamas or vests with poppers to help your child keep their nappy on at night, you can also check out Rackety's (www.disabled-clothing.co.uk), which has a range of suitable clothes as well as draw sheets.

Sleep systems

If your child's ability to move is compromised, they may benefit from a sleep system. A sleep system provides posture control and support for your child while they sleep. If your child doesn't move themselves at night they may be prone to pressure sores. Some children experience breathing difficulties if in a poor position. Other children are prone to muscle contracture and a sleep system can assist in the management of this issue, reducing deformity and pain. A sleep system should assist pelvic stability, trunk and head alignment, and leg positioning. As children are still growing, maintaining good posture has extra importance for their long-term development and comfort.

Sleep systems use a variety of materials including foam or plastic supports to hold your child in a comfortable sleeping position. Some may have Velcro straps, some have covers to assist with temperature-control and pressure issues, and you may want a cotton or sheepskin cover for the sleep system. Your therapist can advise on the best system for your child. There are a number of brands of sleep system. Ask your child's therapist for recommendations and NHS availability.

If your child has profound or complex needs and you are concerned about their safety at night, check out Safespaces (www.safespaces.co.uk). The Safespace is designed for those with autism, epilepsy, challenging behaviour and profound multiple learning difficulties, including those with full mobility. It provides an extremely robust space that can be kicked, punched and headbutted. It can withstand the roughest treatment by both children and adults. It provides a space in which someone can sleep, move, roll or play without restraint, reducing the risk of injury by eliminating hard surfaces.

Funding for equipment

There are a number of charities that can assist families in need of help with funding for equipment:

- ✓ The Tree of Hope offers hope to the families of sick children in the UK who need specialist medical surgery, treatment, therapy and equipment in order to free them from suffering, giving a better quality to their young lives. Visit their website at www. treeofhope.org.uk, email info@treeofhope.org.uk, ring 01892 535525 or write to Tree of Hope, 43a Little Mount Sion, Royal Tunbridge Wells, Kent, TN1 1YP. The Tree of Hope also runs Blossom for Children www.blossomforchildren.com, which offers a range of attractive and useful products for children with medical conditions, disabilities and special needs
- ✓ The Family Fund is the UK's largest provider of grants to low-income families raising disabled and seriously ill children and young people. It helps ease the additional pressures families face by providing money towards essential items such as washing machines, fridges and clothing but it can also consider grants for sensory toys, computers and much-needed family breaks together. There is guidance about how to apply online at www.familyfund. org.uk. First-time applicants can print off a form to fill in, but if you have applied before you will be able to apply online. You can also get in touch via email: info@familyfund.org.uk, via phone: 08449 744 099 or via textphone: 01904 658085
- ✓ The Cauldwell Trust offers a range of core services. Relevant to this chapter, it provides sensory equipment (as well as mobility aids, therapy, family support and more). It says, 'We don't believe in waiting lists for children. Early provision of equipment can prevent the development of associated health problems, stimulate movement and provide essential physiotherapy. We provide mobility and sensory equipment for disabled children

to enable them to live fulfilled and happy lives.' Visit www.caudwellchildren.com where you can apply online or download an application form and apply by post. If you have any questions call the applications helpline on 0845 300 1348.

Summary

There are a few simple actions that will help you make your child's bedroom a place that encourages sleep. Take a moment to assess what might keep them awake, be it light, noise, the temperature or lots of tempting activities.

Declutter the bedroom to make it easy to clear up each night and put tempting toys out of reach. Remove distracting electronic toys, games and the TV. If you can't remove the television from your child's room, cover it up as a sign to your child that it is sleep time.

Make sure that your child is not too hot or too cold at night. Check that their room is dark enough to encourage sleep too. You may also want to look at eliminating any sounds that can interrupt your child's sleep. Check that your child's pillow and mattress do not need replacing. It can be helpful when thinking about redecorating to look at the colours used in your child's bedroom and pick some scents to create a totally restful environment. Organizing your child's bedroom to create a relaxing environment is a positive step to helping them sleep better.

For children with disabilities, illnesses or additional needs, there is also a range of specialist equipment available that can assist with a better night's sleep. Speak to your child's specialist for advice on what will help them. Some help will be available on the NHS, while you may need to pay for other products. There are some charities that will assist with the cost of specialist equipment. See the resources section for a list of full contact details.

Chapter 7
Changing Bedtime Behaviour

In this chapter we discuss behaviour that children may display at bedtime and how to manage behaviour more effectively. Dealing with challenging behaviour can be incredibly stressful and this is intensified if you are feeling tired. We also explore strategies for keeping calm when the going gets tough that tie in well with the following chapter, which covers tips for making bedtime more relaxing.

When you are dealing with sleep issues and a child with special needs it can be incredibly difficult to remain positive. In this chapter we examine the importance of a positive approach to bedtime and positive-behaviour management techniques. We look at how to appropriately reward children's behaviour and what to do when their behaviour isn't acceptable.

Is it an issue?

The first question that you need to examine very carefully is: does your child's bedtime behaviour present an issue?

Do you find that:

✓ You dread bedtimes?
✓ You or your child's anxiety level rises at bedtime?
✓ Your child is adversely affected by lack of sleep the next day?
✓ Your child's behaviour has an impact on your sleep?
✓ Your relationship is beginning to suffer?

If you answer 'yes' to any of these questions you may wish to consider addressing the problem.

If, however, you and your child aren't affected by their unconventional sleep patterns then ask yourself why you are seeking to change the behaviour. Sleep practitioner Emma Sweet explains:

" *Sometimes parents feel that they should change things at bedtime to fit in more with other people's belief systems. For example, one family were very happy co-sleeping but felt that family members were judgemental about this decision. If you are happy with the way things are then you should not feel under any pressure to change it unless somebody is at risk in some way.* "

Sarah recalls:

" *I was asked by a health visitor to attend a meeting for a family of seven children. When I arrived the parents were clearly not aware that I had been invited. It turned out that the health visitor viewed the children's night-time behaviours as being problematic while the family were quite happy with the situation. I explained to the family the service that I could offer but made it very clear that it was their choice. They decided they were perfectly happy to carry on as they were.* "

It is important that you identify the behaviours that you do want to change and that you are committed to making changes as it can be incredibly hard work! Children often resist new boundaries being put into place and this can mean that their behaviours escalate at bedtime. Many parents see this as a sign that the new boundary isn't working when in actual fact it is.

Samantha has a 5-year-old son who had challenging behaviours around bedtime. She says:

" *I'd tried in the past to make changes but always gave up because it was so hard and I felt that I wasn't making any progress. I worked with a sleep practitioner who explained to me that sometimes the behaviour may get worse before it gets better but to stick to using the same strategy consistently for at least two weeks to give it a chance to work. That was the best piece of advice that I was ever given because she was right. My son did resist the boundaries at first and so his behaviour did get worse but this time I had been expecting it so I was prepared. I didn't view it as a failure but as a sign that the boundaries were having an impact. After around a week things started to improve; he stopped kicking off when bedtime approached and became much more accepting of the new routine and boundaries that were in place.* 》》

Bedtime battles

It is important to view bedtime positively rather than as a battle-ground. Some parents feel that the evenings have become a daunting time where power struggles take place and very often they end up on the losing side. It is important to recognize that many children may resist going to bed because there are seemingly far more interesting ways of spending your time when you are a child, including winding your parents up! Some children may feel that they are missing out on something, others may want to continue with pre-bedtime activities and some may simply find it entertaining to watch your reaction as you try desperately hard to get them to go to sleep.

If you have read the previous chapters and eliminated other reasons for your child to resist going to bed including medical issues, pain, fear or anxiety and you feel that the problem may be behaviour-related it is important to identify the trigger for the behaviour. This is something we will explore in detail over the following pages.

One of the first things to do is to make bedtime positive. Have high but realistic expectations of your child and praise them when they meet these. If your child understands explain to them simply what it is that you want them to do.

It is important to recognize that children do overstep the bounda-ries as part of their learning process. And some children need to 'learn' to fall asleep and sleep through the night. For children with additional needs it can take longer to learn these skills. Sometimes it can be about teaching them over and over again simple strategies to help them to fall asleep more effectively.

Sleep associations

We all have associations related to the onset of sleep. For example, in order to fall asleep easily you may need to rest your head on two pillows, and you may need a darkened and relatively quiet environment. If you share a bed with a partner, you may need to sleep on a certain side of the bed. Clothing may be important too, you may need to wear a certain item of clothing such as a night shirt in order to feel relaxed. If anybody removed one of these conditions you might find it harder to fall asleep. So imagine, for example, that I took away your pillows tonight. You would undoubtedly find it much more difficult to nod off. Or what if I insisted you sleep on the floor rather than your usual comfortable mattress?

These sleep associations are relatively easy to keep in place all night. The problem arises when children develop sleep associations that are difficult to maintain. Some children, for example, develop a sleep association around having a parent present. They can then only fall asleep when that parent is there and when they come to a point of waking in the night find that they can't re-settle themselves because they need the parent back *in situ*. Some children require physical contact such as rocking to sleep, again this cannot be maintained consistently throughout the night and so children often wake repeatedly.

Other sleep associations that children may have include:

✓ Night lights – often parents switch these off when they go to bed which means that the conditions have changed and a child will find it hard to re-settle. Imagine if you went to bed in the dark and then someone switched the light on while you were asleep. When you came to a point of awakening you would be highly likely to wake up and protest!

✓ Light shows/mobiles – often these resources switch off once the child has gone into a deeper sleep. If a child learns to go to sleep with this condition in place, however, they may demand it after each sleep cycle

✓ A bottle/milk – some children use milk or a bottle to suckle on as a comforter and then each time they wake they need to be fed back to sleep. This can impact on children's teeth aside from the sleep issues that it may cause

✓ Comforters/dummies – if a child needs a comforter to get to sleep then they are highly likely to need it to be available once they rouse. If it is no longer there then they may well fully awaken

Spend some time considering your own child's sleep associations.

Checklist: does my child have sleep associations?

Ask yourself the following questions:

- ✓ Does my child need specific props in place to fall asleep such as a parent or a soother?
- ✓ Do they get out of bed in the night and move to a different environment to go back to sleep?
- ✓ Do they need it to be light or dark?
- ✓ Do they need sound/silence to fall asleep?
- ✓ Is it important to my child to wear certain nightwear at bedtime?

All of these answers will help you to establish what your child's sleep associations might be and may help you to understand more about their night-time behaviours. The advice that is contained throughout these pages will show you how to make positive sleep associations that are easy to maintain. Where your child already has a sleep association that is causing an issue you can follow the advice around reducing exposure to the association gradually. This will help them to develop a more appropriate association. In some cases you may be able to explore different ways of giving your child access to their sleep association as these two case studies demonstrate:

Laura is a little girl with sensory issues and was moving from her bed to the floor during the night. This was upsetting her parents who repeatedly got up to put her back in bed. James, her father, tells us, 'There is something just not right about seeing your child sleeping on the bare floor. It used to really upset us as parents and we couldn't understand it as we had bought her a lovely new bed that was comfortable and cosy. We contacted the Children's Sleep Charity who helped us to look at things from a different point of view. We explored what it was about the floor that she was seeking out. Well, first of all it was cool on the floor and she is always a warm child. Then secondly Laura seems to like firm touch. She enjoys having her back scratched and will seek out a firm hug; the floor was firm and her mattress was soft. We soon realized that she had developed a sleep association with having firm touch and that her previous mattress had been firm. We recognized that her sleep need was to have firmness and therefore got her a different mattress and so far she has stayed in bed!'

Sam also has sensory issues and learning difficulties. His bedtime routine always involved his parents rocking him to sleep. As Sam was getting older he was becoming increasingly heavy to rock. One of the problems was that Sam would wake frequently during the night and the only way to get him back to sleep was to start the rocking action once more. His parents were exhausted! Donna, his mother, tells us, 'It seemed fine to rock Sam as a baby and a toddler and I just thought that he would grow out of it but he didn't. We got to four years old and were still rocking him to sleep and rocking him throughout the night. I started to suffer with back and shoulder problems as a direct result as he is a solid little boy. We knew that we needed to break the sleep association gradually and took advice around his sensory needs. We use a swing a couple of hours before bedtime with Sam so that he still gets that lovely rocking sensation that he likes. We then decided that it was time to stop the rocking and to get Sam to fall asleep without the motion. It was incredibly difficult at first. I stayed by Sam's bed and gently patted him in the beginning. After a few nights we stopped the patting and I just put my hand on him. We gradually moved on to me sitting with my hand by him and then to sitting by the bed and gradually moving out towards the door. I'm not going to say it was easy because it wasn't but Sam was not distressed as he knew we were there while he learned his new self-settling behaviour. It was tiring carrying this through and I'm glad we did this while we were both on holiday from work otherwise I would probably have given in! Sam has learned now to go to sleep without any rocking and sleeps through most nights. It has been life-changing for us as we used to dread bedtimes. I'm so glad that we took some positive steps to resolve the issue as it was starting to impact on every aspect of our functioning and Sam was an irritable little boy. Even his teachers at school have noticed a difference in his functioning now that his sleep issues have been resolved. And as a couple we are much happier, in fact baby number two is now on the way!'

ABC charts

Sometimes it is hard to work out what may be causing a sleep problem. ABC charts are often used to record daytime behaviours but may sometimes be a useful system for recording night-time behaviours too.

Overleaf is a grid that has been filled in. The 'A' stands for 'antecedent' which simply means 'what came before the incident'. Typically antecedents might include a child being told that it's time to end an activity or parents saying goodnight and leaving the room. Identifying the antecedent is important as it helps us to work out what might be triggering behaviour at bedtime.

The 'B' stands for 'behaviour' and is the section where you explain what behaviour you observed. This could be things like refusing to get into bed or getting out of bed repeatedly.

The 'C' stands for 'consequence' and outlines what happened as a result of the behaviours. This might include things like the child being told off or given a warning.

A (Antecedent)	B (Behaviour)	C (Consequence)
Jack was asked to tidy up	Threw toys everywhere and screamed	Was given a warning which didn't work
Jack was told to go to the bathroom	Refused and lay down on the floor	Was carried to bathroom
Jack wanted one more story	Shouted and screamed	Read one more story to him
Mummy said 'night night' to Jack	Shouted and banged on the floor for Mummy to return	Mummy returned but this continued for two hours

You can now use the blank chart to make your own recordings. Try recording behaviour in the hour leading up to bedtime as well as any night-time behaviours so that you get a full picture of your child's behaviour.

It is also useful to record examples of compliant behaviour so that you can analyze why in certain scenarios your child does comply. Sometimes our children cannot tell us why they are behaving in a certain way so charts such as this can be helpful in supporting us to interpret their behaviour.

ABC chart tips
Here are some tips for using the chart:

✓ Record behaviours for at least a week to see any patterns
✓ Record positive behaviours too
✓ If you can't see what the triggers may be then share the information with a practitioner to see if they can help you to make more sense of the information
✓ Be honest!
✓ Make a note of days and times to see if behaviour is influenced by daytime activities

A (Antecedent)	B (Behaviour)	C (Consequence)

Behaviour management strategies

The strategies that you use to manage your child's bedtime behaviour will very much depend on their cognitive ability. Some of the strategies suggested below may not be appropriate due to your child's individual needs. As a parent you are the expert on your child and you should use your judgement to decide what may work well.

Language

For children with learning difficulties language can be confusing. It is important to think about the way that you give instructions to your child. Do they understand what you are asking of them? Use sign-supported materials if necessary, such as a visual timetable. Use your child's name to gain their attention and if they can verbalize check that they have understood what you have asked them to do.

The 'when then' rule

The 'when then' rule can be incredibly effective when working with children who want to be in control. Saying to a child 'when you have eaten your supper you can then have your toys' is much more motivating than saying 'you are not having your toys until you have eaten your supper'.

Here are some more examples of the 'when then' rule turning negative instructions into more positive instructions:

✓ 'When you have tidied your toys away, then we will have a story', rather than, 'I'm not reading you a story until you have tidied your toys away'

✓ 'When you have turned the television off, then we will make a picture', rather than, 'Turn the television off or I'm not making a picture with you'

Think about ways that you can use the 'when then' rule to make choices more positive at bedtime.

Mind your manners

Rather than saying 'please' try using 'thank you'. If you say to a child, 'Turn the computer off please' it suggests that it is a request. If you say, 'Turn the computer off, thank you' it suggests that they don't have an option and that you expect it to be done. Using 'thank you' also gives the impression that you trust them to do what you have asked which can be very motivating for a child.

Choice-making

Most children like to feel like they are in control and want to make choices. Choices can be offered for many things at bedtime such as:

✓ Which story would they like to hear?
✓ What would they like for supper?
✓ What toy would they like to play with?
✓ Which bath toy would they like tonight?

Children can be offered visual choices so actually holding out two story books and asking them to choose can be helpful. It can also underline the fact that you are only reading one of the books tonight. Choice-making is good for non-verbal children and they can be encouraged to make a choice through eye-pointing or reaching out if appropriate.

Ignoring

Sometimes negative attention can be better than no attention at all in a child's view. Consider whether the way that you deal with things at night-time is the best way.

Claudia has a son, Isaac, who is nine years old. She says:

" *Isaac had never slept well and I was at the end of my tether to be perfectly honest. I look back now on how I used to be at night-time and cringe. I was so tired and worn out that I realize that the way I reacted to him getting up in the night wasn't appropriate. I used to shout at him and try to reason with him, saying things like, 'Mummy needs to be up for work in three hours and I just can't function.' He wouldn't have a clue what I was talking about but it almost made me feel better to verbalize it at him. Looking back, I can see that he was getting attention, albeit negative attention, from his night-time behaviours. In Isaac's world it was better to see me even if I was ranting like a mad woman, than to not see me at all!* "

Sometimes ignoring behaviour can be an appropriate behaviour-management strategy, particularly in the run-up to bedtime. If, for example, a child throws a toy do you need to intervene? Most children do want to be noticed. You could try telling them that once they've picked the toy up then you will help them and turn away from them to give them the chance to conform. Or for other children simply ignoring the behaviour may give them a chance to modify it and then you can acknowledge them when they do the right thing.

The important thing about using ignoring as a strategy is that you need to immediately reward your child with your attention once they do comply. It is not safe to ignore some behaviours and you should be mindful of this.

The broken-record technique

The broken-record technique is a positive-behaviour management strategy than can prove extremely useful at night-time! This involves parroting back a set phrase to your child to give them a clear signal that at night-time you are not entertaining! You should choose a phrase that you would like to use such as 'It's night-time, go to sleep' or simply 'It's sleep time'. This should be the only phrase that you use during sleep hours, unless of course your child is ill or has had a nightmare or so on.

The great thing about the broken-record technique is that it helps you to stay in control of your emotions. You know exactly what you are going to say and it avoids you getting angry even though you are feeling tired. You need to be persistent in the use of this technique and use a calm voice.

Sue says:

> *I was taught the broken-record technique on a sleep workshop and it was the one thing that really helped to save my sanity. I realized I'd been bargaining with my child during the night and actually that was utterly ridiculous. At times I'd also been cross and genuinely felt anger towards her which again is not a good place to be. I used a set phrase from putting her to bed and then parroted it during the night. I was a bit sceptical about it to be honest as I didn't see how it would work but I was desperate to try anything. At first she tried to push me to say something else by throwing more and more behaviour in my direction but gradually it did get better. One thing I will say about the technique is that it helped me to feel more in control. I felt calmer just by saying my set phrase. I realized that my daughter had become in control at bedtime and this simple strategy actually helped me to regain control which was empowering in itself.*

Liaison with school

If your child has behaviour issues in the daytime then they are highly likely to have behaviour issues at night-time too. It may be useful to speak with your child's school or pre-school to establish strategies that they use when dealing with this issue. It is important that behaviour is dealt with in a consistent manner. It is also useful to highlight to the school that you are working on a sleep programme and to see whether they are able to offer any support via trained family support workers.

Positive reinforcement

It is important that you do praise positive night-time behaviours just as you would daytime behaviours. In this section we will explore different ways to positively reinforce behaviours at bedtime.

Using praise effectively

We all like being praised and it is important to maintain a child's self-esteem. Here are a few tips about using praise effectively:

- ✓ Be specific about what you are praising so don't just say 'good boy' as that is meaningless. Say things like 'I like the way you listened to your bedtime story so nicely'
- ✓ Be sincere with your praise
- ✓ Don't use it as a bribe but use it because you are genuinely pleased that your child has achieved something
- ✓ Be consistently positive

Focus on the process of bedtime so pick out small elements to praise initially such as having a positive bath time. If you are going to use a reward system it is important that you set your child a small and achievable target. It is important that your child sees some success otherwise they will become demotivated so ensure initially that they do receive regular rewards. You then need to make the rewards more challenging to gain. Rewards should never be used as a bribe. For example you should never say, 'If you go to bed now I'll give you a star'.

Rewards are a positive-behaviour management strategy and therefore you should never take a reward away once it has been given. If you do take it away it becomes a negative strategy and you will find your child will become demotivated. Consider this scenario to understand how it may feel for a child to have rewards taken away. Imagine that you have worked hard all week and on the Friday you get paid appropriately. The following week you make a mistake and the manager decides to take all your wages from you. How do you feel?

Children are motivated by different things and below we will explore some ideas for rewards. You may need to review the reward system that you use on a regular basis to ensure that it continues to be motivating for your child.

Reward charts

Reward charts can work effectively for some children and can be a positive way of rewarding good bedtime behaviour. Your child needs to be able to understand the concept of reward charts in order for them to work.

If you are going to use a reward chart make sure that it is on display where your child can see it. Be consistent in offering the rewards on the chart. Sometimes it may be necessary to add in another motivator, for example, when the chart is full a small treat can be gained such as a comic or action figure – whatever motivates your child.

Individual rewards

Some children do not respond well to stickers or reward charts and need more specialist rewards that motivate them. Think about what your child loves to do and whether you can encompass this in a reward system. Sally has a son aged eight who has learning difficulties. Here she tells us about his reward system:

“ *Seamus has never been one for stickers or reward charts; they just don't interest him at all. One thing he loves though is sea-shells. He enjoys touching them and holding them to his ear to 'listen to the sea'. We have been down the route of reward charts to no avail so I started to think outside the box. I decided to make him a reward box and in there are all sorts of different shells. It has been brilliant because he is so motivated by it. For him this is a reward worth having whereas he is likely to eat a sticker!* ”

Dealing with night-time behaviours

There are only a few different ways to deal with a child's behaviour during the night. The thing about all of the methods is that in order to work they need to be used consistently whichever method you choose. These methods will only work if used alongside a good bedtime routine and an appropriate bedroom environment.

Controlled crying

Controlled crying is often used as a sleep-training method for infants to teach them to self-settle. Many parents feel uncomfortable using this technique as it involves leaving children to cry while checking on them after certain intervals of time.

When using controlled crying you return to the room five minutes after you have left to briefly check on your child. Your reappearance is designed to reassure your child that you are still there. If you are going to use this method then you should not offer comfort to your child but tell them to go to sleep. You then increase the time before you reappear by another five minutes until you are checking on your child only at fifteen-minute intervals. The idea is to continue this until your child falls asleep. The procedure is then repeated every time your child wakes throughout the night.

There is lots of conflicting research around controlled crying with some researchers suggesting that it can lead to youngsters feeling stressed even once they have fallen asleep. Other research suggests that it is a perfectly safe technique to use and will not cause any psychological damage. For parents of children with additional needs it can be a highly stressful method to use as often our youngsters cannot communicate to us what their needs are and it is important that we respond to their needs. If you feel that this is not the right approach for you then there are gentler ways to teach children to sleep through the night.

Gradual retreat

Gradual retreat is a method that usually works well for parents of children with additional needs. If your child needs you to be there in order to fall asleep then this is a good way of teaching them to fall asleep without you but in a gentle way.

If you are currently lying down with your child then you may move a little further away such as sitting on the bed or sitting next to the bed. The idea is that you will move away physically over a period of time. Your child is highly likely to try to get you back into their bed so it is important that if you choose this approach you remain consistent. Do not interact with your child while you are in their room and stick to a set phrase if you need to say anything at all such as, 'It's sleep time'.

We've all tried to tiptoe out of our child's room only for them to wake up. In order to ensure that you can successfully leave the room you may need to wait until they've been asleep for around ten minutes. If your child wakes up during the night you need to go back to the point that you were at while they were asleep. Some parents find that it is easier to move a mattress into their child's room to sleep on while they are working on a gradual retreat programme.

This is a gentler programme than controlled crying and it can take longer for your child to learn to fall asleep independently using this approach.

Rapid return

Rapid return can be used successfully for children who get out of bed repetitively. This technique involves returning the child to bed without engaging with them. If your child will not stay in bed then this may be a technique that you could consider. Initially you may want to stand outside the door so that you are in place to return your child as soon as they try to leave their bedroom. The key with this approach is to remain consistent and not to give the child attention for their behaviour.

It is likely that your child may also get out of bed in the middle of the night and again you need to use the same technique of taking them back to their room quickly and without offering them any reward. For some children a reward can be being picked up by a parent so if at all possible try to lead them by the hand.

Summary

It is important to remember that most sleep issues are behavioural but if you are unsure you should seek professional advice to rule out any medical reasons. With behavioural issues they are likely to get worse before they get better and knowing this before you embark on a sleep programme is very important.

The key to success with behavioural issues is to remain consistent in your approach. This can be extremely challenging when you are sleep deprived yourself but is also incredibly important.

Use an ABC chart to work out what might be triggering certain behaviours that you would like to change. Read the section on behaviour management and think about the words that you use, as well as the way you respond to negative behaviours. Work out what positive ways you can praise good behaviour and reward your child.

Get support networks around you if at all possible to help you through this process, and keep sleep diaries so that you can review your progress. Once we start on sleep programmes it is very easy to lose sight of how successful interventions are. A sleep diary should be reflected on at least weekly so that you can see the progress that you are making as a family.

Chapter 8
Promoting Relaxation

In this chapter we explore the important role that relaxation plays in the bedtime routine. Many of the parents that we have spoken to during our research for this book described the run-up to bedtime in negative terms. One mum described it as 'stressful and chaotic' while another referred to it as 'an utter nightmare'. Children with additional needs tend to pick up on parental stress levels and a stressful lead-up to bedtime is not conducive to a good night's sleep.

It's important that we look at strategies for keeping our own stress as parents well managed even when things don't go to plan. It can feel impossible to find time to relax when you are the parent of a child with additional needs so we will find out how other parents in similar situations manage it. We also explore different methods of relaxation to try with children in order to encourage them to wind down before bed.

Many children with additional needs also suffer with anxiety issues. It is important that these issues are acknowledged and managed in an appropriate manner so that they do not unnecessarily hinder sleep. Over the following pages, we hear from experts in the field as they share strategies to try and also explain when professional help should be sought.

Fear of the dark and separation anxiety are also discussed in detail. This chapter is packed with case studies from parents who have found successful strategies for coping with bedtime stress.

Stress and bedtime

There is no doubt about it, being a parent can be incredibly stressful. Parenting a child with additional needs also brings a whole range of extra pressures to your life and when your child doesn't sleep household tension can rise to crisis point.

Miriam says:

" *I can't tell you how stressful night-time is in our household. I can feel my stomach begin to tighten as bedtime approaches. By the time I actually get Jenny into bed I'm either ready for shouting or ready for crying. I then get cross at myself for getting into such a state but I'm just constantly on edge, waiting for her to start screaming. I'm looking at the clock and wondering how much longer she is going to be awake for and how much sleep I will manage to get. By the time I do get to bed I am so wound up that even if Jenny is asleep I can't then nod off. It's like a vicious cycle.* "

Sadly Miriam's story is not unusual; when we are sleep-deprived we are less likely to cope well with stress. Children with additional needs pick up on non-verbal signals and if you are feeling stressed throughout the bedtime routine the chances are that your child will pick up on this stress and start to feel uptight.

The symptoms of stress

Stress can present with different symptoms depending on the individual. It is important to listen to your body and monitor your stress levels. Symptoms may include:

- ✓ Shaking
- ✓ Headaches
- ✓ Heart racing
- ✓ Mouth ulcers
- ✓ Asthma
- ✓ Panic attacks
- ✓ Poor sleep patterns
- ✓ Inability to concentrate
- ✓ Irritability

Debbie tells us, 'I was actually under a consultant at the hospital for constant migraines. I'd had scans, medication, you name it. Once my son's sleep problem was resolved I found that the migraines disappeared. I believe they were a symptom of being chronically stressed and sleep deprived.'

Sleep deprivation and stress can leave us with many side effects as Debbie's story has demonstrated.

Managing stress levels

If you are concerned about your stress levels you should book an appointment with your GP. Always seek medical advice if you are concerned about your health. It is also important that you explore positive strategies to manage your stress more effectively.

Claire has a daughter with complex needs and sleep issues. She advises parents to seek out others who understand.

" I find talking about my situation helps me to relax and calm. I do however have to find the right people to talk to. Many people simply don't understand how hard it is to parent a child with additional needs who doesn't sleep well. It annoys me when people try to help and say things like, 'Have you tried putting her to bed a bit later?' or 'Have you tried giving her a glass of milk before bed?' What is helpful is when I phone my friend up and she listens to me and really hears what I say. She has a son with similar difficulties and she understands how difficult life can be at times. I also find parenting groups can be a good source of support too. I think people have to have experienced the situation to really understand how it feels and what it is like. "

Talking about your situation can most certainly help to reduce stress. If we feel supported we are more able to work out a strategy to manage our difficulties more effectively. To find out about local support groups contact your local family information service which is based within your local authority.

Other parents find that they can gain support online from people that they may never have met in real life. Sally says:

" I use parenting forums that are specifically for children with additional needs. I find that the parents there are more

understanding than the more mainstream forums. The good thing about these is that even if you are up in the middle of the night you can generally find another parent to chat to; this helps to stop me feeling so alone. When you are the only house in the street with a light on at 3 a.m. you can feel as if you are the only person in the world going through these difficulties. I've also gone on to meet up with a lot of the parents in real life and made some great friendships. "

Building support networks can be incredibly important for some parents and can help them to manage stress more effectively. If you think that it would help to talk to other parents you may wish to consider contacting Scope; they run a befriending service called Face2Face. The service puts you in touch with a trained parent befriender who can offer emotional support. Details can be found on the website at www.scope.org.uk.

Sometimes it can be helpful to change the way that you think about the situation. If when bedtime begins to approach you think 'this is going to be terrible', the chances are that you will have a really stressful evening. If there are points in the run-up to bedtime that are challenging remind yourself that they will not last forever and that you can handle them because you have done before. Also, be kind to yourself; praise yourself when you have done a great job.

When changing sleep habits in children it is important that you are realistic. Don't set yourself targets that are too high or you will feel downhearted if you don't reach them. Make sure that you celebrate any targets that you do meet. As parents we are very good at criticising ourselves for what we perceive that we have done wrong but we aren't as good as giving ourselves a pat on the back for all the things that we have got right. Reflect back on the sleep diary if it helps and look at how your child's sleep patterns are improving over time. Celebrate even small achievements; think of them as building blocks for improved sleep in the future.

It may be that you only feel like you can make small changes to your child's sleep routine at the moment because life is difficult and making a bigger change feels too daunting. If this is the case make small, manageable changes and praise yourself for recognizing your limits and not attempting too much at once.

The importance of relaxation for parents

Relaxation time is important for everyone because it helps us to deal with our stresses more effectively. When we feel tense our bodies release the hormone cortisol in what is referred to as the 'fight or flight' response. This leads us to breathe more quickly, our heart will race and adrenalin will be released around our body. Our body can be placed under a great deal of pressure and it is important that it has a release through relaxation so that these effects can be reversed.

Relaxing can, however, be particularly challenging if you are a parent with a child that doesn't sleep well. In this section we will explore some tips that other parents have tried to promote relaxation around their children.

Dee says:

I always thought that I didn't have time to relax but what I've come to realize is that I must make time to relax otherwise I will burn out and won't be able to look after my family. I've had to learn to say 'no' to some things such as a friend asking a favour. That was a difficult lesson to learn as I was so eager to help everybody but I've realized that in order to continue to be effective as a mum I need to make time to relax myself.

Scott is dad to Joel, aged twelve. He says:

I felt guilty having any 'me time' until recently. I realized that I was becoming worn out and depressed. My GP suggested I take part in some form of exercise to help with my stress levels. Being a single dad to a child with special needs, it isn't easy to get out and about to do this, so I bought an exercise bike. I make sure that I use it every other night and I actually look forward to these sessions now. I feel more positive and I'm feeling fitter too.

There are a number of relaxation techniques that you can try at home. Relaxation techniques can take practice and it is important that you make time for yourself so that you can carry on caring for your family. If you learn to relax your body your mind will follow.

Breathing exercises are very helpful in promoting relaxation. When we are stressed we breathe more shallowly which leads us to feelings of panic. Practice breathing deeply when you have a few moments, your inward breath should be shorter than your outward breath ideally. Breathing in for the count of seven and out for the count of eleven is useful. This is something that you can practice discreetly at any point in the day and when bedtime approaches and you begin to feel uptight remind yourself to breathe the stress away.

Sue says:

" *I used to get really panicky at bedtime and I'd find I would start to feel faint. I realized after attending a sleep workshop that it was all down to my breathing. I've started to carry out breathing exercises now to help me to stay calm and I'm really surprised by the results. Also, if I do start to feel jittery, simply counting while I breathe helps to take my mind off the situation too. It acts as a welcome distraction. I'd recommend that other parents give it a go.* "

There are many products on the market that you can buy to help you to relax at home. You may wish to explore meditation as a way of helping you to wind down, or hypnotherapy; CDs are available to buy or you can download material online. Carol says:

" *I'd always thought hypnotherapy was a load of rubbish to be honest until my friend trained to become a hypnotherapist. I was still very sceptical but then I started to see the results of her work. She gave me a relaxation CD to listen to at home and I have to admit I found it very relaxing. I now listen to it every few nights, it really does help me to calm down and I find I sleep better too the night that I've used it.* "

Some parents find that taking up a new hobby is also helpful. Jayne enjoys card-making and says, 'I find that I just need something for "me". Being a full-time carer to a youngster who doesn't sleep very well can be highly stressful. Card-making lets me lose myself for a little while and I find it incredibly relaxing. It is also something I can do without leaving the house which is an added bonus.'

The importance of relaxation for children

When we are in a relaxed state we are much more likely to benefit from a better night's sleep. Marneta Viegas is the director of Relax Kids and a leading expert in child-relaxation techniques. Marneta explains:

Relaxation is vital prior to bedtime as children's bodies and minds need time to unwind from the day. If children don't have time for relaxation they may fall asleep but the sleep may not be as restful. Children are inundated with information and it is becoming increasingly necessary to give them the opportunity to take time out to be quiet and still. Relaxation can help the overactive, anxious and stressed mind; teaching simple relaxation techniques to children can give them tools that they can use throughout their life.

Marneta believes that children with additional needs can learn to relax. 'Teaching children with additional needs relaxation techniques takes time, patience and consistency. Initially a group of children with autism that I worked with were unable to sit still for more than a few seconds; they are now taking part in regular relaxation sessions lasting up to twenty minutes, and most importantly they love it.'

It is important that when you are working with your child to promote relaxation that you are calm yourself. Prepare a calm atmosphere to work in. You may wish to consider using blankets, cushions and soft music in the background. Turn off the television and telephone ringers; it is important that the environment is tranquil. Begin with short sessions initially to get your child to engage and gradually extend the length of the sessions as they begin to enjoy them more.

Ideas to promote relaxation

Marneta has some relaxation exercises from Relax Kids to try with your child. You will need to consider your child's skills in order to choose a relaxation activity that is appropriate to their individual needs. Some children with more profound and complex needs may appreciate listening to calm music while enjoying a hand massage; other children may be able to engage in these more imaginative ideas.

'For children who feel anxious or tense at bedtime you can encourage them to tighten all their muscles as tight as possible and then to relax them. Ask them to notice the difference and how they felt when the muscles relaxed. Pay particular attention to the shoulders and the jaw.' This would be a good one for parents to take part in too.

Children can also be taught breathing exercises. Marneta says, 'If your child is able to imagine that there is a butterfly on the chest ask them to do so. Tell them, "Each time you breathe in and out the butterfly will gently rise and fall again, breathe in and breathe out."'

Teaching children positive self-talk can also be a good tool. Marneta suggests telling children:

> *Repeat to yourself 'I am calm,' 'I can stay still'. Some children will respond well to music, encourage them to dance and move quickly and then let them lie down still as soon as the music stops. Extend the periods of lying down so that children get used to lying still for longer periods. Don't worry if your child is not able to concentrate and keep still for very long, the most important thing is that you are creating new habits and positive patterns.*

For those children who can engage with a longer visualization exercise, Marneta has kindly written the following to be shared with your child. Encourage your child to lie on the floor and play some soft, gentle music in the background:

At the beach

We are going to lie on a warm beach. It will be warm and quiet, the sun will be shining. You will lie on soft, warm sand. You will see soft, white, fluffy clouds as you look up. You will be able to hear the soft gentle waves lapping against the shore. You will feel very warm and relaxed at the beach. You will feel calm and relaxed and safe at the beach. (Pause and possibly take a deep breath yourself.)

I will count to twenty very slowly. (Pause, music still playing.)

You will close your eyes, lie quietly and listen. (Long Pause.) One, two, three, you can feel your body on the floor. You can take a long breath in and out, again. Four, five, six, you feel warm and comfortable, breathe, seven, eight, you can feel the warm soft sand under your back, nine, ten, you can feel the cool breeze blowing gently over your face. The air is cool and fresh. (Pause for a longer time).

Eleven, twelve, thirteen, the sun is shining, making you feel warm. You can hear the calming sounds of waves lapping against the shore. You can hear the soft wind blowing. You can hear the gentle sound of seagulls flying in the distance. Fourteen, fifteen, the sun is shining over the water, you see small white clouds moving slowly across the sky, you can smell the salt in the air. Breathe in gently and breathe out, breathe in, breathe out, sixteen, seventeen, eighteen. You feel warm and calm, you are comfortable and safe. (Pause.)

Nineteen, twenty – you are lying on the soft sand on the beach. You are quiet. You feel warm. (Long pause).

Relax, the sea is relaxing, the sun is warm, you are going to relax and lie still. You are lying on a warm beach. You feel warm and comfortable. You can feel the cool breeze blowing gently on your face. You feel warm and relaxed. (Pause.)

I am going to count you back. I will start at twenty, when I get back to one you will be in back in the room feeling calm and relaxed. Twenty, nineteen, you are lying on the soft sand on the beach. You are quiet. You feel warm. (Long pause.) Relax, the sea is relaxing, the sun is warm, you are relaxed and lie still, eighteen, seventeen, sixteen, you feel warm and calm, you are comfortable and safe, fifteen, fourteen, the sun is shining over the water, you can see small white clouds moving slowly across the sky, you can smell the salt in the air, breathe in gently and breathe out, breathe in, breathe out, thirteen, twelve, eleven, you still feel warm. You remember the sounds. You begin to be aware of sounds around you. You are relaxed. Ten, nine, the warmth of the sand has made you relaxed. Your body is feeling relaxed and supported by the floor. Your breath is gentle. You feel calm, eight, seven, six, five, you are beginning to slowly move your fingers. (Pause.)

Now slowly move your toes. You can hear your breathing in and out. Four, you feel calm and comfortable, three, two, one, breathing in and out, you will slowly and quietly open your eyes. You are back and you feel calm and relaxed. When you are ready you will slowly get up as relaxation has now finished.

Anxiety and sleep

If your child is anxious it may hinder their sleep. When youngsters are sleep deprived the physical symptoms associated with anxiety tend to intensify. It is important that you seek professional help if your child's anxiety levels are impacting on everyday life. However, there are strategies that you may wish to consider trying at home to help to manage your child's anxiety levels more effectively.

If your child tends to be a worrier it is important that they are given a positive way of dealing with their worries so that they may feel some release from them. Worry boxes are a good way of encouraging this. A worry box can be made from any cardboard box and decorated with some wrapping paper. A slit should be put in the top and your child encouraged to write down any worries that they have. If they don't have writing skills they could draw a picture or mark-make a symbol to represent their worry. Once they have done this they simply post it into the worry box. This strategy may be useful for those children who wake in the night with a worry.

Worry dolls are another useful tool to help to manage worries more effectively. These lovely little colourful dolls originate from Guatemala and children who cannot sleep tell their worries to them.

For younger children blowing their troubles away can be a useful introduction to simple breathing exercises. Encourage a child to blow their troubles through a straw into some water to make them into bubbles.

Talking is a great way of releasing anxiety. Spend some time in the early evening talking about how the day has been and if there is anything worrying your child. Always plan these sessions well away from bedtime as you want your child to have time to have discussed their worries and moved on from them.

Ending the day positively

Positive language makes us feel better and helps to program our minds in a more positive way. Ending the day in a positive way can be helpful to generate a better night's sleep. Irene says, 'Callum made me smile when he asked me to tell him that he would have a good night's sleep with lovely dreams. I asked him why I needed to say this and he told me because he would then have a good night's sleep with lovely dreams and he did.'

Talk about the lovely things that have happened at the end of the day rather than any worries or concerns. You may wish to talk about what is going to happen tomorrow that is wonderful. End the conversation by telling your child one thing that you are proud of them for today and reassure them that they will have a great night's sleep.

Fear of the dark

We know that it is helpful for children to sleep in darkened environments to support their melatonin production but some children are generally frightened of the dark. Firstly it is important to acknowledge that most children do express fears of the dark at some stage. Consider the matter from your child's point of view; see what they see from their bed at night. Sometimes it can be that car lights on the road outside cast shadows that may be frightening if they are left unexplained. Or maybe it is a dressing gown hanging from the door which looks frightening in the darkness. Don't be dismissive of the fear; acknowledge that you understand that they are afraid and that you will support them to overcome this fear.

There are lots of children's story books that help to normalize fear of the dark. Ask at your local library for recommendations. You may wish to consider using a night light which gives off a soft glow throughout the night to offer reassurance. Or if appropriate you could put a torch by the side of the bed so that your child can switch it on if they do become afraid. Touch lamps can work well too and are relatively easy to operate.

Separation anxiety

Some children can become anxious around separating from their parent; they may not understand that you will be returning for them. Sometimes giving a child a transitional object can be useful. Sarah says:

66 *Matthew used to be desperately upset when I said goodnight to him. No amount of reassurance helped. I worked with a sleep practitioner who advised giving him a cotton handkerchief and telling him that it was my special object. I put the handkerchief under his pillow and asked him to keep it safe for me and I'd collect it in the morning. It worked a treat! He seemed to understand that I would come back for the handkerchief if not for him!* 99

Other ideas include putting a T-shirt that you have worn over the pillowcase. This may help children to smell your natural scent and reassure them that you are still around. Some children find it helpful to have a photograph of their parent by the bed.

Bath time

As we discovered in Chapter 5, bath time can help to promote a better night's sleep. A warm bath can encourage the release of melatonin which helps children to fall asleep more easily. What you need to consider is whether your child finds having a bath a relaxing experience. If they do then make sure you include it as part of their wind-down time. If they find it stressful or they become excited at bath time it may be better to keep it out of the bedtime routine.

Complementary therapies

More people are turning to complementary therapies in order to promote relaxation. You may find that using a complementary therapy such as reflexology or massage helps you to manage your stress levels more effectively.

Sian has a reflexologist visit her at home, 'When you have a child with a disability it is incredibly difficult to find time to relax. I enjoy reflexology and treat myself to regular sessions. It fits in with my daughter's needs as the practitioner can visit me at home. I find that I feel more relaxed after the sessions and I really do look forward to them.'

Seeking further help

If you feel that your child's anxiety levels are not improving despite consistently trying strategies to promote relaxation you may need to seek more specialist advice. You should share your concerns initially with a medical practitioner such as your GP, paediatrician or health visitor.

Dr Louise Langman is a chartered clinical psychologist and sees children with additional needs and sleep issues. She tells us:

In my role as a clinical psychologist, settling and night-waking problems seem to be the most common. When families have tried over long periods to alleviate the issue a number of compounded impacts can occur – parents become sleep-deprived themselves and totally exhausted, often their capacity to maintain collaborative and satisfying relationships with their partners can deteriorate due to having different ideas about how best to tackle the problem. Over time the quality of the child-parent relationship may also suffer. If siblings do not have sleep problems, the child who does may be blamed and scapegoated. Where there is just one child, parents may demonstrate resentment since their once satisfying relationship has been lost. Clearly the impact of sleep problems is wide-reaching not least for the child themselves.

Dr Langman explains that while some children have sleep issues from birth others may be triggered by more specific events or even a series of events such as separation from a primary caregiver or a change in routine. She goes on to say:

> *Psycho-social factors associated with getting off to sleep and waking in the night can include parent-child attachment difficulties and parental anxiety or depression. When there is a secure parent-infant attachment the parent will allow the infant enough time alone when settling or during night-waking episodes to allow the child to 'self-soothe' and return to sleep. Where an anxious infant-parent attachment has formed the parent may not leave the child alone for long enough before sleep or during a night-waking episode for the child to develop the self-soothing skills required.*

Dr Langman explains:

> *Reassurance for the child that their bedroom is a safe place and that nightmares are only dreams is appropriate but by the time the problem is serious enough to warrant a clinical psychology referral, it is unlikely that simple reassurance will be of benefit. Usually these experiences will be occurring as part of a broader response to a life situation that involves threat to the child's safety, security or self-esteem. Threats may include moving house, changing school, parental separation, parental hospitalization, the birth of a sibling, car accidents, burglary, bullying, physical, sexual or emotional abuse. Bedtime fears and nightmares often reflect the child's attempt to process and gain control over bewildering or frightening features of their current life situation.*

Where appropriate, the clinical psychologist will work with the parents to listen to their child's fears, facilitating their expression and empathizing with them. Dr Langman says, 'I often teach parents how to help their children learn relaxation skills by modelling within the session. The child will be helped to process their feelings, the parent and child will be encouraged to overcome any avoidance in talking about issues and the role of facilitative parent as a "secure base" will be strengthened.'

Clinical psychologists are employed by the NHS and work in multi-disciplinary teams within Child and Family Services or Child and Adolescent Services. You can seek referral to your local specialist team by meeting with your GP or paediatrician. Alternatively, to directly contact a clinical psychologist in your area, log on to the Association of Child Psychologists in Private Practice www.achippp.org.uk. It is essential that your clinical psychologist is registered with the Health Care Professions Council (HCPC) and is chartered with the British Psychological Society. You can check their qualifications by logging on to the HCPC website www.hpc-uk.org/check/.

Summary

It is important that at bedtime the household is a calm and relaxed place to be. Stress and anxiety can affect you, the parent, and make bedtime doubly hard. Stress will also impact on your own sleep, health and well-being. Some children need help to learn to relax: anxiety is associated with some specific additional needs.

Sometimes we need to spend time focusing on learning to relax and this is a particularly important skill to teach children. Many of the activities that we have suggested in this chapter can be shared activities and you and your child can enjoy relaxing together.

Start with short lengths of time and build on these gradually. Make sure that you persist with whichever relaxation activity that you have chosen as it can take time to see results. Ensure that whatever activities you choose for both yourself and your child they are motivating. Relaxation time should be enjoyable for you all.

Chapter 9
Specific Additional Needs

Introduction

In this chapter we will explore the impact that specific additional needs may have on a child's sleep. We will also look at what you can do practically to help improve your child's sleep issue and who you can turn to for further support.

Read this chapter to find out more about the sleep issues and solutions that are associated with:

- ✓ Autism
- ✓ ADHD
- ✓ Down's syndrome
- ✓ Cerebral palsy
- ✓ Learning difficulties
- ✓ Visual impairments
- ✓ Hearing impairments
- ✓ Angelman syndrome
- ✓ Kleine-Levin syndrome

Autism

Children with autism often have sleep issues; in fact, sleep problems seem to be more common in these children than in the rest of the population.

There can be a number of reasons why these sleep issues occur. Sleep is a very difficult concept to understand; some children with additional needs may be fearful of falling asleep: how do they know that they will wake up? What happens to them when they are asleep? Children with autism can be very literal in their thinking and this can impact on their anxiety around sleep.

Emma Sweet at the Children's Sleep Charity gives us an example:

> " *I set up a visual timetable for a child who is on the autism spectrum. I recognized that he would benefit from having the routine visually on display. The last symbol on the timetable showed a child in bed. The little boy followed the timetable and got into bed; he couldn't understand that he then needed to go to sleep as the child on the timetable wasn't asleep! I then changed the timetable to show that the child was asleep in bed, thinking that this would work. Unfortunately this didn't work either as the timetable showed a child going to sleep but nothing afterwards. This caused the little boy some distress. I then had to add a 'waking up' symbol to the chart so that he could clearly see that he would wake up and to show the full cycle. Sometimes we forget that the children we are working with are so literal and that the things that we say may cause them to be confused or even distressed.* "

Social cues can be missed which means that children with autism may be less likely to pick up on the signals that bedtime is approaching. Visual timetables can be helpful for some children to encourage them to learn and follow the bedtime routine.

Social Stories are also a useful tool to encourage children to learn about bedtime in a positive manner. They were introduced by Carol Gray who has a wealth of experience in working with children on the autism spectrum. The stories have become recognized as being a highly effective way of introducing children to social and life skills, particularly when they are on the autism spectrum. Social Stories guide children through basic activities and help them to understand why they take place. They can be used effectively to help children understand the different aspects of bedtime. As adults we don't always consider things from our child's point of view and may not realize how stressful bedtime can be. To read more about Social Stories and Carol Gray's work visit www.thegraycenter.org.

Although children with autism tend to enjoy routine they often develop their own bedtime routine that may not be in line with the rest of the family's. Tim tells us about his son who is now ten years old.

    " *Ben loves routine but his bedtime routine was very much on his own terms. He used to like to stay in his room and watch specific programmes and then play on his PlayStation. Prior to bed he had to line up all his toy cars and if one was in the 'wrong' order that would cause a meltdown. If we tried to intervene he would get distressed and aggressive. It was really hard implementing a new routine. We had to do it a little bit at a time and give lots of reassurance along the way.* "

For children on the autism spectrum sleep time can provide them with a perfect opportunity to take part in their own more self-directed activities. For children who can't cope with social pressures night-time can provide a perfect environment where they can pursue their own interests uninterrupted. John is eighteen years old and has Asperger's syndrome. He tells us:

    " *I like to be up in the night; it is quiet and I hate noise. I am tired in the daytime now and know I can't concentrate well on my exams; this is making me anxious but my favourite part of the day is night-time. I look forward to everyone going to bed and being able to be alone, doing my own thing.* "

Sensory issues are commonly experienced by children on the autism spectrum. Having issues with touch, visual stimulation and sound can present an additional challenge when it comes to going to sleep. An environment can easily seem over-stimulating to an autistic child. Some children find it helpful to have a low-arousal workspace at school and likewise a low-arousal bedroom environment.

    Children with autism can be particularly sensitive to allergies and food intolerances. It is worth keeping a food diary to see whether you can work out any links between diet and sleep patterns. See Chapter 4 for more on food diaries.

Some children are also sensitive to fibres so it may be worth exploring the different types of mattresses and duvets available on the market as some are more suitable for children with allergies than others.

Some children with autism respond well to using a weighted blanket at bedtime. Sue King, spokesperson from Kingkraft, explains about them:

A weighted blanket is an effective way to apply weight and deep pressure which has been found to be both calming and comforting for some individuals. The weight and deep touch pressure to the body stimulates the proprioceptive sense, enabling those who are 'sensory seeking' to relax by improving their body awareness. The proprioceptive sense gives us information about our body's position and movement via receptors in our skin, joints, muscles and ligaments. Children with poor proprioceptive sense have difficulty processing these sensations which often result in behaviours that give them sensory feedback, e.g. jumping, running, spinning and chewing. As a result these children often have problems sleeping as they find it difficult to 'switch off'.

Sue goes on to explain:

The weighted ball blanket, in addition, stimulates the touch sense via touch receptors on the skin to help neutralize an under- or over-responsive tactile system. By lowering anxiety levels it brings about a sense of calm and an improved sleep pattern.

There has recently been new guidance issued over the use of weighted blankets following a tragedy in Canada where a child was swaddled in a weighted blanket and died. Weighted blankets should be used under the guidance of a therapist and a risk assessment should be carried out. The blankets should never be wrapped around a child but placed on top of the child like a duvet. See Chapter 6 for more about weighted blankets.

There have been a number of research studies that suggest that children with autism do not produce enough melatonin. It is extremely common for children to be prescribed melatonin in order to help with their sleep though you can use other methods to increase melatonin production naturally such as:

✓ Limiting screen activities for the hour leading up to bedtime
✓ Dimming the lights in the hour leading up to bedtime
✓ Giving a warm bath if appropriate half an hour before bedtime
✓ Using blackout blinds in the bedroom to create a dark sleeping environment
✓ In contrast, ensuring that your child is exposed to natural daylight each morning

See Chapter 4 for more about melatonin.

The National Autistic Society has a section of their website dedicated to advice around sleep issues. Visit www.autism.org.uk.

ADHD

Children with a diagnosis of ADHD are also highly likely to have sleep issues. Children with ADHD are more likely to suffer from daytime sleepiness, habitual snoring and restless legs syndrome than other children. Bed-wetting is also more common in children with ADHD than in other children. Interestingly, children who are sleep deprived are more likely to display hyperactive behaviours and be more challenging. Lack of sleep can certainly make the symptoms of ADHD worse.

If you suspect that your child may have restless legs syndrome or sleep apnoea you should seek medical advice. A behavioural approach to managing children's sleep problems can be extremely useful. One study found that eliminating sleep issues by using a cognitive and behavioural approach eliminated hyperactivity and attention issues for some children.[22]

It can often take children with ADHD a long time to fall asleep at the start of the night. Some research suggests that children with ADHD release melatonin later in the evening by around two hours, resulting in them being awake for longer and not becoming tired until later in the evening.

Many children with ADHD find it difficult to switch off in order to go to sleep. The fact that they may be aware that the clock is ticking and they are expected to be asleep can fuel anxiety, which in turn makes it harder to nod off. The chapter on promoting relaxation, Chapter 8, will be useful to encourage children with active minds to use their brain in a different way to promote relaxation and calm at bedtime. A good bedtime routine is essential with regular wake-up times incorporated to encourage the strengthening of the circadian rhythm.

Waking up can be particularly challenging for children who have fallen asleep late. Alarm clocks that wake users gradually by filtering light into the room may be useful to ensure that waking is not done suddenly: this can cause distress. For older children, having a number of alarm clocks may be necessary to ensure that they do wake up and don't go back to sleep.

If your child is taking medication be sure to check the side effects. Some medications used to manage ADHD can actually be stimulants and increase sleep issues. Discuss the issue with your child's medical practitioner; sometimes moving the dose further away from bedtime can be helpful. See Chapter 4 for more about medication.

Samantha has a daughter aged twelve who has a diagnosis of ADHD. She tells us:

❝ *Sophie's sleep patterns have always been poor and caused us issues. She just doesn't seem to get tired and is always on the go. At night-time she will stay awake until the early hours but then struggles to wake up for school. I used to get cross with her but now realize that this is all part of her condition. One of the things we did find is that what she does before bedtime has a direct result on the amount of sleep she gets. We swapped the computer for calmer activities which she didn't like initially but we stuck to our guns and it did pay off. We also tweaked her bedtime. I worked with a sleep practitioner from the Children's Sleep Charity and realized that there was no point putting her to bed at 8 p.m. when she wasn't falling asleep until 11.30 p.m. Sophie was getting stressed and we were getting stressed. So we put her to bed at 11.30 and then gradually moved her bedtime by fifteen minutes every three nights. I was reluctant to try the idea at first as it seems wrong putting a young child to bed so late but it was explained to me that her own natural body clock was out of synchronization and it needed readjusting gradually. We also had to get her up at a set time each morning, that was tricky too. We did notice a great difference though and she went from sleeping at 9 p.m. to 7 p.m. in the space of a few months.* ""

Sophie says, 'I don't dread bedtime any more. I used to get wound up and the more I thought about going to sleep the more I couldn't go to sleep. Now it's a lot easier to fall asleep and I feel better too. I'm doing better at school and my teachers have noticed a difference in my work, I'm really pleased about that.'

If your child is accessing services via your local CAMHS team be sure to tell them about the sleep issues. It is possible that they have a sleep practitioner working within their team and that they are able to offer you support around improving the sleep issues.

Down's syndrome

Children with Down's syndrome are also particularly susceptible to certain sleep issues. It may be that the issues are physical, behavioural or a combination of both. It is useful to keep sleep diaries and to share these with the practitioners involved in your child's care in order to ascertain whether your child's issues are behavioural. If so, children with Down's syndrome respond well to a structured bedtime routine where they are taught how to fall asleep independently.

Simone was ten years old when her mother decided it was time to tackle her sleep issues. Here Tracey speaks honestly about why it took her so long to address the issues and how she found it:

ɛɛ *When Simone was a baby I was incredibly protective of her, particularly as she has Down's syndrome. I used to rock her to sleep and worried about her constantly. She was never a great sleeper but I read that children with Down's syndrome don't sleep well so I accepted that this was part of her condition and something I'd have to get used to. The years went by and Simone still didn't sleep well; she would need me there in order to fall asleep and then would be up frequently in the night. I researched using a behavioural programme at bedtime and parents spoke really positively about it. I decided to find out more and met with the sleep practitioner. It worried me when she said it may get worse once I put boundaries in place and I didn't feel like I could cope with that. I decided to wait a few months before starting the programme so that I could get myself in the right mental state to keep at it. I did and within a month Simone's sleep patterns were greatly improved. There were no tears while carrying out the programme either, it was gentle and she responded well to the boundaries in place. I wish I'd done it years ago now as she is happier in the daytime and I'm happier too.* **ɟɟ**

Choosing the right time to implement a sleep programme is key and Tracey was quite right to wait until she felt that she was in a better place to carry out the work. Children with Down's syndrome can take longer to learn new skills and it is just the same with sleep. They may take longer to learn the associations with bedtime and it is therefore important that we remain consistent when dealing with their behaviours at night-time.

Children with Down's syndrome are more at risk of having Obstructive Sleep Apnoea (OSA) than other children. It is possible that OSA exists alongside a behavioural issue around sleep too. Healthcare professionals should be informed if your child has sleep issues and they should investigate whether the difficulties are physical, behavioural or a mixture of both.

Enlarged tonsils and adenoids in children with Down's syndrome make them more likely to suffer from OSA. A referral to an Ear, Nose and Throat specialist may be required or you may consider requesting a sleep study where a detailed assessment can be made. If your child sleeps in an unusual position then you should also mention this. Sometimes children adopt different sleeping positions to try to open up their airways. If your child does get bunged up with mucus it may be helpful to avoid the usual advice of offering a glass of milk at night-time. Dairy products can increase mucus secretions which is not helpful for children with Down's syndrome, as their facial structure tends to mean that their airways are narrower.

Cerebral palsy

There are a number of reasons why a child with cerebral palsy may suffer with sleep issues which may include:

✓ Difficulties with digestion
✓ Problems with disordered breathing during sleep
✓ Discomfort due to muscle spasms
✓ Medical factors such as epilepsy impacting on sleep
✓ Learning difficulties, which make it harder to learn a bedtime routine
✓ Sensory impairment
✓ Constipation

Where there are multiple professionals involved in a child's care it is important that a multi-agency approach to sleep is taken. The physiotherapist is best placed to offer advice around comfort and appropriate sleep systems. Sleep systems can be custom-made to suit your child's needs and to ensure that they are in a comfortable position at night-time whilst supporting their posture. Read more about sleep systems in Chapter 6.

An occupational therapist can offer support around the sensory issues affecting sleep while a paediatrician can input to ensure that any medical reasons for the sleep issue are managed as effectively as possible. A behavioural approach to sleep is still highly likely to improve a child's sleep patterns and the advice in the book around improving sleep hygiene should be followed.

Sharon's daughter has cerebral palsy and has never slept well. She tells us:

❝ *Kirsty is thirteen now and has always had problems sleeping. I accepted that it was due to her additional needs and never really thought to address it. I then met another mum at a support group who had a child with similar needs; she told me about using a behavioural approach to sleep and I was keen to learn more. I enrolled on a sleep workshop and met other parents who were going through similar issues; that helped me to feel less alone. The tips that were offered were really good and doable. I recognize that sometimes Kirsty will wake up because of discomfort but actually I think some of her wakings were due to the fact that she had never learned to fall asleep independently.* **❞**

Sharon goes on to explain the importance of sticking to the routine:

❝ *I was determined to have a go at setting a good routine and at sticking to it. It was really difficult and I was exhausted while carrying it out but Kirsty responded well to the new night-time boundaries that I put in place. I acknowledge that she doesn't need as much sleep as some of her peers as she isn't as physically active. I also acknowledge that she will wake in the night on occasions due to her physical needs. This has taken some of the pressure off me to be honest as I now work with her needs rather than reading parenting books which talk about typically developing children and highlight the differences even more. I think the best advice I can give other parents and carers is to be open minded about trying new things. I thought that Kirsty would never be a sleeper but she's proved me wrong, yet again!* **❞**

If there are 'Team Around The Child' meetings already taking place for your son or daughter then do bring up sleep as an issue. If these meetings aren't in place but you think that they would be useful you can suggest to the practitioners involved that you wish to initiate these so that everybody involved in your child's care can meet on a regular basis.

Learning difficulties

Sleep problems are frequently reported by parents of children with learning difficulties. It can take children with learning difficulties longer periods of time to learn what is expected during the night-time. Parents often get support to manage daytime behaviours while at night-time they are left unsupported.

Sometimes a child may have neurological issues that impact on their sleep. If this is possible, it is important to always seek medical advice. A sleep study may also be helpful to find out more about the difficulties that your child is experiencing.

It is important to remember that when a child has learning difficulties we have to reinforce boundaries repeatedly; it is the same at night-time. It can take children with learning difficulties longer to learn about falling asleep independently or what to do if they wake in the night. It is important to keep language simple, just as you do in the daytime. Consistency is extremely important so that your child learns what to expect. Children with learning difficulties thrive on routine and enjoy knowing what will come next so a good bedtime routine is vitally important to help them to feel secure at night-time.

Visual impairments

Sleep problems are more common amongst individuals with significant visual impairments. Visually impaired children with no perception of light may have difficulties distinguishing night from day, which can then impact on their circadian rhythm. For these children it is important that other cues are built into the bedtime routine, such as music to indicate the time of day. Sticking to strict bedtimes and getting up times is also helpful to keep your child's natural body clock well tuned. For children with visual or hearing impairments melatonin can be helpful to support their circadian rhythm and help it gain a more established pattern.

For those children with limited sight, putting them in a bedroom environment with blackout blinds can be disorientating. Here Sally talks about how her daughter's difficulties cause distress when she is in total darkness:

" *Sophie is visually impaired but does have some sight. I'd read about how important it is to put a child in a dark environment to sleep and that's what I did. Sophie used to get very distressed during the night. Her specialist teacher explained to me that it may be too dark for her with her limited use of vision. Actually I was completely taking away her vision which made her feel anxious and she then wasn't sure where she was when she was waking up. I now use blackout curtains which provide a dark environment but not as dark as the blinds, I always leave a gap in the curtains too to let a little light filter in. She's been much happier and slept better since I made these little changes.* "

Hearing impairments

Children with hearing impairments may be more at risk of sleep issues. They are certainly at risk of having some disturbance of their circadian rhythm. Melatonin may be considered in order to support the body clock but it is also useful to follow a bedtime routine. Using visual clues to aid your child's understanding about the passing of time is key. Make sure the environment is dark at night and light in the morning. If appropriate, use a clock to reinforce timings. If your child cannot read a clock then stick symbols onto a clock to show when key events will take place.

Tinnitus can cause a buzzing sound in the ears which can be distracting at night-time. Researchers have, however, found no link between the loudness or pitch of sounds associated with tinnitus and the presence of sleep disturbances. Nevertheless, sound therapy systems can be purchased that may be useful, the idea being that they play nature sounds which can help to ease the tinnitus.

Angelman syndrome

Sleep problems are very common amongst children with Angelman syndrome. There may be behavioural difficulties at night-time combined with difficulty getting to sleep and frequent night-time waking. Many parents worry about the safety of their child when they are getting out of bed during the night. If safety is a concern you should speak with an occupational therapist about risk assessing your home and your child's night-time behaviours. Door alarms may be helpful, as may investigating a Safespace sleep system for your child.

If your child tends to get very warm it may be worth thinking about their clothing at bedtime. Breathable bedding can help to let heat escape and may be worth exploring. Many children respond well to a structured bedtime routine too.

Kleine-Levin syndrome

Kleine-Levin syndrome (KLS) is a rare syndrome characterized by bouts of excessive sleep of fifteen to twenty-two hours daily for days, weeks and sometimes months at a time. The sleep is accompanied by reduced understanding of the world and very marked changes in behaviour.

The signs of KLS are of a teenager (or more rarely a younger child) who is sleeping for unusually prolonged periods of time. The teenager is completely exhausted, uncommunicative, does not understand what is happening and is not behaving as usual. They often complain of de-realization (where nothing feels real). They are confused, unable to concentrate or communicate and they appear childlike, apathetic (with little or no facial expression) and sometimes they can carry out repetitive behaviour (such as watching the same television programme over and over again). They often have a grey pallor with dark circles around the eyes. Sometimes they eat compulsively or act in a disinhibited way. They often complain of migraine headaches and they are hypersensitive to light and sound. Sometimes they can struggle to maintain a regular body temperature. If prevented from sleeping, they may become anxious and irritable. Apart from the three core symptoms of excessive sleep, cognitive impairment and altered behaviour, other symptoms may vary. Indeed, symptoms can vary within each episode of KLS. The child may be in an episode for days, weeks or even months. In between these episodes they will return to usual sleep, cognition and behaviour, but they will have little or no memory of the period they have missed.

Jane's experience of KLS began when she could not wake her 12-year-old son. Here she explains what happened:

❝ *When he eventually got out of bed at 1 p.m. after seventeen hours in bed he appeared to be sleepwalking. He had terrible headaches which no medication helped, he would not wash or get dressed. He ate excessive amounts of food in a mechanical fashion. When not sleeping, he watched the same television programme over and over again. Although usually sporty, sociable and happy at school, he would not leave the house. After five months he woke up and he had no memory of the previous five months during which he had been ill, but he was keen to see friends and return to school and his normal life. He was then well for seven months until the following year when he again had the same symptoms for five months.* **❞**

Polly was an outgoing, sociable 17-year-old student when she suddenly complained of her head feeling strange and nothing feeling real. Within twenty-four hours she had an excruciating headache which no medicine helped and she could not physically stay awake. She slept for twenty-two hours a day for almost three weeks. She had no expression on her face, she was upset by light and sound and she just wanted to be alone in the dark in her room. She did not appear to understand when her mother spoke to her. She did not want to eat or drink and had to be forced awake to drink fluids. Polly also did not want to wash or dress. After three weeks she woke up and she was desperate to return to her normal life. She had no recollection of what had happened over the previous three weeks. During the next year she had five more episodes of varying length totalling 104 days. After the initial few episodes, some of Polly's symptoms changed – she slept for twenty hours a day and when awake she had an insatiable appetite, craving unusual, sweet or salty food. When awake she appeared childlike, sucking her thumb, cuddling a soft toy and wanting to be close to her mother. She became anxious if her mother left the room. She watched the same children's fairytale film over and over again. When each KLS episode ended she returned to her normal life as a college student.

The cause of KLS is currently unknown. Some children's first episodes are accompanied by a virus. No specific tests can be carried out and a diagnosis is made through a clinic interview with the child and their family after the exclusion of other conditions. The average length of time for a diagnosis of KLS is four years. KLS Support UK is a small charity offering help to those affected by the syndrome. If you would like help or advice contact: www.kls-support.org.uk.

Further support

If you are concerned about your child's sleep patterns it is important that you get appropriate support in place. You should discuss your concerns with your child's medical practitioners to find out whether any support is available in your locality. Some local authorities buy in specialist sleep services that have sleep practitioners who can offer you one-to-one support. If you are worried about your child's sleep you should seek immediate medical advice via your child's GP or paediatrician.

Below are a number of charities who may be able to offer you further support:

The Children's Sleep Charity cover England and Wales and offer support to families who have sleep issues. They are specialists in working with families of children with additional needs. You can find out more about their work by logging onto their website at www.thechildrenssleepcharity.org.uk.

Sleep Scotland's vision is, 'that all families of children and young people with additional support needs and severe sleep problems in Scotland can be helped to achieve a qualitative improvement in the whole family's life, and that this service should be provided in partnership with the statutory sector'. You can read more about their work at www.sleepscotland.org.

Cerebra provide sleep support for families of children with brain related conditions. Cerebra's spokesperson, Elaine Collins, tells us more:

❝ *Cerebra provides a free service to parents of children up to sixteen years old who have a neurodevelopmental disorder or brain injury and who are experiencing sleep deprivation. The service aims to support parents by raising awareness about quality sleep and why it is essential. We work to educate parents and help them to gain a better understanding of why their child may be experiencing poor sleep. The team can empower and support parents and carers to manage their child's sleep by offering possible solutions that can be implemented and tried.* **"**

Elaine goes on to explain how the service is delivered:

" *The sleep service can offer parents face-to-face support through sleep clinics or home visits. To date we have sleep counsellors available in the south west, Wales, the central region, the north west and the north of England. Additionally we can give advice by telephone, post or email.*

The sleep service also works to raise awareness amongst professionals about sleep disorders and their management and we can give presentations and workshops.

Cerebra has a series of information factsheets on a number of issues which are available free from our website. **"**

Information factsheets currently available from Cerebra include:

- ✓ Bed-wetting
- ✓ Good sleep hygiene
- ✓ Nightmares
- ✓ Night terrors
- ✓ Anxiety at night
- ✓ Night-waking
- ✓ Sleeping alone
- ✓ Rhythmic movement disorder
- ✓ Biology of sleep
- ✓ Melatonin

To access the leaflets and to find out more about the service log on to www.cerebra.org.uk.

Scope's Sleep Solutions service offers sleep practitioner support in some localities as well as workshop training for parents and practitioners. To read more about the service log on to www.scope.org.uk.

Chapter 10
Planning Intervention

In this chapter we consider how to address your child's sleep problems in a way that you feel is manageable. We look at how you can interpret data that you may have built up through observation and sleep diaries. We also share with you examples of good bedtime routines and case studies from families who have successfully managed to improve their child's sleep patterns.

As we have emphasized throughout this book, if you are unclear as to whether your child's sleep issues are behavioural or medical you should always seek advice and guidance from a medical practitioner. It is vitally important that medical issues are ruled out before taking a behavioural approach to sleep. However, implementing good sleep hygiene is important for all children and should always be used alongside medical treatment to promote a better night's sleep.

Looking after you

It might sound silly to ask 'how are you feeling?' when you are suffering from sleep deprivation but when you are sleep deprived you can feel a lot more than just tired! Sleep deprivation can have a devastating effect not only on your mental health but also on your physical health. Individuals with sleep deprivation can often feel depressed, have weakened immune systems and find it difficult to function on a daily basis.

Take five minutes to think about how you are feeling and jot your feelings down below. We've added a few ideas to get you started:

I am feeling . . . .

✓ Exhausted
✓ Frustrated
✓ Angry

It is important that you acknowledge your feelings. If you are in a relationship it is also important that your partner is aware of your feelings and vice versa. You could ask your partner to complete the same exercise to find out exactly how they are feeling. You may have similar feelings, but don't be surprised if sleep deprivation affects you and your partner in different ways. Sleep deprivation can impact significantly on relationships. Acknowledging this is an important step.

If you find that you are having negative thoughts and are even feeling depressed you should speak to your GP. Talking about these feelings is important. Often we feel that we should be able to cope and keep feelings bottled up.

Lynn Wilshaw is a Relate counsellor. She tells us:

❝ *Sleep problems can lead families into crisis. Single parents are already under a great deal of pressure and can find that sleep issues on top of parenting alone can have a devastating impact on their lives. For those parents that are in a relationship, sleep issues can cause significant difficulties. Lack of sleep can cause us to snap at our partners and feel low, and may cause resentment if one parent feels that they are left to deal with the issues. Parents' sex lives can also be adversely affected by lack of sleep which again may cause relationship issues. Acknowledging how you feel is important and speaking about your situation can help, either to friends or family who are non-judgemental or to a counsellor.* ❞

The Relate for Parents and Families website has a facility for a live chat with a Relate counsellor. You can chat about any aspect of family life that is causing you difficulties and the consultation is free and confidential. To find out more about the service log on to www.relateforparents.org.uk.

Siblings and intervention

There is no doubt about it, when you start a new sleep programme it may impact on the sleep of all the other household members. It is a good idea to consider when would be a good time to start the programme based on each individual's needs. If you have older children trying to concentrate on exams, for example, it would be better to wait until the exam period is over before making any changes.

It is likely that your other children's sleep is already affected by the sleep issues in your household. Make sure that you let the school know what is happening at home as disturbed sleep can impact on a child's ability to learn and concentrate. Hayley is a teacher and says:

    I can definitely tell which children in my class are sleep-deprived. Those children find it much harder to concentrate and to learn. It is important that teaching staff are made aware of any sleep issues at home as we can then deal with things in a more supportive manner. It is a very different scenario if a child is awake at night due to the sleep issues of a sibling compared to if they choose to be awake playing computer games.

If at all possible try to arrange things in the house so that any siblings' sleep is disrupted as little as possible. Consider whether their bedroom is the most appropriate to meet their needs. Some families have temporarily turned a dining room into a bedroom to give their child a much-needed restful environment whilst carrying out a sleep programme. If your children share a room then it may be that you need to think creatively about erecting partitions within that room to minimize disruption. It may be worth exploring whether a relative can accommodate the sibling for occasional nights too, to ensure that they get some level of good sleep.

Listening to your other children is extremely important. They need the opportunity to talk openly and honestly about how they are feeling. It may also be helpful for them to know that you are looking at ways of addressing the issue as you do recognize the impact that sleep issues are having within your family. Ask your child if there is anything that they can think of trying that might help to support them to get a better night's sleep. It is important that they feel included in decisions that are made and that they recognize that you are trying to improve things. If your child would find it helpful to talk to others then Sibs is a charity that represents the needs of siblings of disabled people. They can provide information and support around living with a sibling who has a disability. You can find out more about their work through their website at www.sibs.org.uk.

The right time

Before you begin work on resolving your child's sleep difficulty it is important that you identify the most appropriate time for you as a family to work on the problem. Sleep problems can be challenging for parents and carers to address and you need to have the right support in place around you.

Is it the right time? A handy checklist

You may wish to consider the following:

✓ If you are working would it be better to book some annual leave while you are implementing changes?
✓ If you have other children who may have their sleep interrupted how will you manage this?
✓ What support networks do you have in place around you and how can you utilize these?
✓ Is there a practitioner involved in your child's care who can support you with making the changes?
✓ Have you got a period of time that is uneventful to implement this? It's a good idea to avoid implementing a new routine prior to a holiday or Christmas, for example

Consistency is key

Once you decide that you are going to make changes it is important to remain consistent in your approach. Dedicate two weeks to each strategy in order to ascertain whether it is successful. Many parents implement a strategy and when their child resists it they think that the strategy doesn't work. In actual fact, they needed to keep consistent for longer to see the true results.

Dr Andrew Mayers is a senior lecturer in clinical psychology and statistics at Bournemouth University. Dr Mayers has a specialist interest in sleep. He recognizes that it can be incredibly difficult for parents to change sleep issues and offers the following advice:

Be aware of the need for change, and recognize that it may require everyone in the family to make changes, not just the affected child. Also, be aware that any changes must be applied consistently, and may take several weeks to take effect. It is unlikely that the required outcome will be seen straight away, so it important to keep the new plan going, even when it seems like it is not working. It is all too easy for parents to become so wound up about their children's sleep that they don't make time to wind down themselves. Parents need to learn relaxation techniques so they give a calm appearance. A calm parent helps to calm the child. Use the child's wind-down time to relax, and put away the stresses that you may have had during the day. Focus with the child on something nice that you have done together. Take the time to read to your child, or ask them to read to you.

To read more about Dr Mayer's work on sleep visit his website at www.andrewmayers.info.

Getting to the root of the problem

Many parents feel overwhelmed with advice in the face of their child's sleep issue. The important thing to remember is that you need to identify what is causing your child's sleep issue before starting to implement any of the strategies that we have discussed. Often there can be numerous factors that impact on your child's sleep rather than just one reason. In this book we have explored many different reasons why children may have sleep difficulties. These reasons can include:

✓ Environmental factors
✓ Sensory issues

✓ Medical problems
✓ Behavioural difficulties

You may find that you have a list of five or six possible reasons that your child's sleep is disrupted. It is important to explore each of these reasons fully.

Thinking about your child's issues, use the table below to write down what these may be and what strategies you could use to address them.

Possible sleep issue	Strategy to try
Example: gets up frequently during the night to play with toys. Over-stimulated during the night? Are there environmental factors affecting sleep? Could medical issues be a problem?	Example: make toys inaccessible at night-time. Make the bedroom environment calm and less stimulating

Strategies to use

The strategies that you use should always be ones that you feel comfortable with. Sometimes it can seem overwhelming when you are trying to tackle a sleep problem, so to begin with just choose one new thing to try. Debbie tells us about her experience:

" *When I started to think about Ella's sleep problems I realized that there were lots of things that might be causing her to wake in the night. For a start she was sleeping in a brightly coloured room with lots of twinkling lights, and she always went to sleep with the television on. Looking back, her bedtime routine wasn't great and I responded to her very quickly so that the rest of the house wouldn't be woken up. It did help for me to break these issues down and to consider how I would overcome each one in turn. At first I felt totally overwhelmed and didn't know where to begin but I started by just making one change: I decorated the bedroom. This was something that actually helped as I could see a physical transformation taking place and a calmer environment being created. It was also good because I could see something for all my effort. After the decorating I felt more motivated to take another step so I decided it was time to move the television out and restrict viewing before bed. Once I'd got this established I started work on a better bedtime routine. It isn't easy but when you break the problem down it really does help you to see things more clearly and it helped me to feel more in control too.* "*

Using sleep diaries effectively

In Chapter 1 we introduced you to keeping a sleep diary. It is important that you use the data that you have collected in this sleep diary to inform which strategies you will use to tackle the sleep problem. The first thing to do is to check the amount of sleep that your child is having and consider whether the number of hours is roughly appropriate. Do remember that children are all individuals and the amount of sleep that they need will vary from one child to the next. The Early Support booklet 'Information About Sleep' provides information about average sleep needs of children and can be downloaded free of charge by following this link: www.ncb.org.uk/media/875230/supportsleepfinal.pdf.

If you find that your child is having the right amount of sleep it may be that their sleep patterns have shifted and that they are having the sleep at the wrong time. So, for example, Peter goes to sleep at midnight and gets up at 10 a.m. This is causing his mother problems as he needs to be at school for 8.30 a.m. The amount of sleep that he is having is reasonable for his age but it takes place at the wrong time. In this case we would advise that Peter's mother puts him to bed earlier by fifteen minutes every three nights and wakes him fifteen minutes earlier every three mornings until his body clock becomes set to a more appropriate sleep time.

If you have a pre-school child then you should also check that their nap times are appropriate and not too close to bedtime. You can implement a nap-time routine to help your child to learn about sleeping during the day.

A good bedtime routine should last no more than an hour. Check your sleep diaries to see how long your bedtime routine takes. Some families develop elaborate routines that can be used by the child as an avoidance strategy when it comes to bedtime. If it is taking longer than an hour then you need to review what you are doing prior to bed.

Examine the sleep diary to see how long it takes your child to fall asleep after getting into bed. If it is taking more than fifteen minutes on a regular basis your child may have a problem with sleep onset and self-settling. If your child doesn't fall asleep for a long period of time after going to bed on a regular basis you may need to review the bedtime routine or timing.

Antony has a son with additional needs and sleep issues. He says:

" *Kieran is five years old and is currently under assessment at our local Child Development Centre. He has never slept well. Keeping sleep diaries was useful for us as a family and what we found is that it can be two or three hours after getting into bed before Kieran falls asleep. We were advised by a sleep practitioner to temporarily alter his bedtime. Instead of putting him to bed at 8 p.m. like we were doing, we were told to put him to bed at 10.30 p.m. as that was when he was showing signs of tiredness. We were horrified at first as our aim was to get him to bed earlier not later. It did help though and we found that we weren't as stressed at night-time. Before we had been going backwards and forwards to him all evening. We found he did fall asleep more quickly with the later bedtime and then we could gradually alter it by fifteen minutes every three nights so that he was soon falling asleep at 8 p.m. without any difficulties. We even managed to pull it forwards some more and he now is fast asleep by 7.30 p.m. We would never have thought of doing this ourselves but it worked!* 🗦🗦

As well as the going-to-sleep time, it is important to look at your child's waking-up time. If they are waking early consider whether they are getting enough sleep. Is it actually a night waking that you are responding to?

Antony explains further:

🗦🗦 *The sleep diaries also helped us to look at the way we were dealing with things. Kieran used to wake up at 4.30 a.m. and we used to take him downstairs so that we didn't wake his brothers up. Actually this was probably just a night waking so we were told to use a set phrase and help him to settle back to sleep. Using blackout blinds also helped to stop the light coming in as much which he seemed to be particularly sensitive to. Dealing with the night waking in this way has meant that they have reduced and virtually stopped alto-gether now.* 🗦🗦

It is important to be clear about what hours are 'sleep time' in your house. Parents are often very clear about what time bedtime is but not as clear on what time is acceptable to start the day. Use the sleep diaries to establish what time your child currently wakes up. If they tend to stay in bed until you wake them, then look at a reasonable time to wake them up and wake them consistently every day of the week, even at weekends! This will help to strengthen their circadian rhythm. If they are waking early in the morning then treat this as a night waking rather than the start of the day.

Planning the routine

In Chapter 5 we discussed bedtime routines in depth. Now it is time to use this information and create a good bedtime routine that your child will respond to.

Decide first of all what time your child will be going to bed; you need to work backwards from here in order to decide when to start your routine. If your child is in bed for 8 p.m. then you should turn screens off at 7 p.m. and plan for this hour in some detail.

Bedtime routine checklist

The things that you need to consider are:

✓ What time will your child eat?
✓ What activities will you do in the hour leading up to bedtime?
✓ Who will put your child to bed?
✓ What set phrase will you introduce?
✓ Will you use music to give a sense of time?
✓ Is a bath appropriate within the bedtime routine?
✓ Will you use a bedtime story?

The template below shows a bedtime routine used for Amy who is twelve years old and has learning difficulties.

Time	Activity
6:45 p.m.	Supper – Amy enjoys a piece of wholemeal toast and a glass of milk
7 p.m.	Turn the television off and dim the lights Enjoy hand eye co-ordination activities such as jigsaws, rolling dough and bead threading Amy uses her visual timetable to choose activities that she wants to engage in. A sand timer is used to warn her that this time is coming to an end and that it will soon be bath time
7:20 p.m.	Amy has a bath

Time	Activity
7:30 p.m.	Pyjamas on, toilet, tooth-brushing etc.
7:45 p.m.	Amy is tucked into bed. The bedside lamp is on and she enjoys a bedtime story
8:00 p.m.	Hugs and kisses from mum and her older brother. State 'It's sleep time now' and leave the room, switching the light off

The template opposite will be useful for you to plan out your child's routine in detail and to share it with others who may put your child to bed. Remember to begin with the time that your child goes to bed and work backwards.

Celebrating success

It is vitally important that you have a positive approach to bedtime. You need to make sure that you celebrate your child's achievements as discussed in Chapter 7. You should consider implementing a reward system that your child will respond to and make sure that you praise them for good night-time behaviours.

It is also important that you celebrate your own success. Parenting a child with additional needs is extremely challenging, and parenting a child with additional needs *and* sleep issues can be exceedingly difficult. Some parents find it useful to keep sleep diaries over a period of time so that they can reflect back over them and see the progress that their child has made. Your support has enabled this progress to be made so never undervalue the role that you have in these changes.

Summary

Identifying why the sleep problems are occurring is extremely important so that you can identify an appropriate strategy to use. Consistency is key in dealing with sleep issues and you really do need to ensure that once you start a programme you are able to follow it through. Celebrating success is vital and you need to remind yourself frequently that you are doing a good job.

Time	Activity

To end on a positive note, Claire is mother of a son with complex needs who did have sleep issues. She tells us:

" I always accepted that Jack's sleep issues were part of his medical condition so just felt that this is how life would be. It wasn't until I heard about using a behavioural approach to sleep that I thought things might be able to be improved. With support from a sleep practitioner I took on board all the advice and was amazed that it worked. Jack now sleeps through most nights. It is my personal experience that led me on to train as a sleep practitioner myself. I'm passionate about supporting other families and want to share the information with them. I am a volunteer for The Children's Sleep Charity and love spending my time empowering other families to make a positive change. "

Resources

The Children's Sleep Charity was set up by co-author of this book Victoria Dawson. Its aim is to offer support to all families who have children with sleep issues. Sleep workshops are offered across England and Wales and training is available for sleep practitioners. The charity hopes to secure funding to offer online and telephone support in the future. To find out more about its work log on to www.thechildrenssleepcharity.org.uk or find it on Facebook.

The Early Support booklet 'Information About Sleep' provides information about the average sleep needs of children and can be downloaded free of charge by following this link: www.ncb.org.uk/media/875230/earlysupportsleepfinal.pdf.

While most of this book is about the sleep issues of children aged between two and nineteen, Isis (the Infant Sleep Information Source) provides information about babies' sleep based on research. The website also provides factsheets around infants' sleep. Read in depth information at: www.isisonline.org.uk.

Support resources for you

If you feel that you need somebody to talk to, you may wish to consider one-to-one or couples' counselling. Your GP is able to make a referral if necessary, or you can contact a private counsellor, although a fee would then be involved.

You may also wish to explore Relate for Parents and Families which is a website that offers support and access to online chat with a Relate counsellor. For more information about this service log on to www.relateforparents.org.uk.

The Parent Partnership Service offers information, advice and support to parents and carers of children with special educational needs. Its role is to support parents in having their views understood and you may be offered support when attending meetings. The Parent Partnership Service is a voluntary organization and provides confidential and impartial advice. To find out more about their role and to locate your nearest service log on to www.parentpartnership.org.uk.

Face2Face is a service managed by Scope and trains parents of disabled children to befriend other parents. If you need some emotional support Face2Face has services across England and Wales and also offers an online service. For more details contact Scope: www.scope.org.uk.

Support resources for the family

Sibs is a UK charity that was set up to support the needs of those growing up with a brother or sister with additional needs. Their website is packed full of useful information about how to support siblings through difficult times. Log on to www.sibs.org.uk.

Specialist equipment and funding

If you need specialist equipment and it is recommended by a professional, ask first if it can be supplied on the NHS. If that is not an option, the internet has made it much easier to shop around for resources. Some useful sites are listed below.

Blossom for Children www.blossomforchildren.com

Easy Blinds for a range of blackout blinds www.easyblindsonline.co.uk

Fledglings www.fledglings.org.uk or read the catalogue at www.fledglings.org.uk/docs/pdf/brochure

The Gro Company: items to support sleep including the Gro Clock, room thermometers, blackout blinds and children's sleeping bags from baby sizes up to age ten www.gro-store.co.uk

Kingkraft weighted blankets www.kingkraft.co.uk

Magic Blackout Blind: statically charged polypropylene film blackout blinds www.magicblackoutblind.co.uk

Promocon: suppliers of continence products www.promocon.co.uk and www.disabledliving.co.uk

Rackety's www.disabled-clothing.co.uk

Relax Kids www.relaxkids.com

Social Stories www.thegraycenter.org

Aromatherapy blends for children www.speciallittlepeople.co.uk

There are a number of organizations that offer funding for equipment. Each has different requirements:

The Tree of Hope offers funding for specialist medical surgery, treatment, therapy and equipment.
www.treeofhope.org.uk
info@treeofhope.org.uk
01892 535525
Tree of Hope, 43a Little Mount Sion, Royal Tunbridge Wells, Kent, TN1 1YP

The Family Fund provides grants to low-income families raising disabled and seriously ill children and young people towards essential items such as washing machines, fridges and clothing, sensory toys, computers and family breaks.
www.familyfund.org.uk
info@familyfund.org.uk
08449 744 099
Textphone: 01904 658085
Family Fund, 4 Alpha Court, Monks Cross Drive, York, YO32 9WN

The Cauldwell Trust provides sensory equipment (as well as mobility aids, therapy, family support and more).
www.caudwellchildren.com
Applications Helpline: 0845 300 1348

More organizations, professional bodies and specialist groups

Association of Child Psychologists in Private Practice, www.achippp.org.uk, 07563 955808

British Association of Occupational Therapists, www.cot.co.uk, 020 7357 6480

Cerebra, www.cerebra.org.uk, 01267 244200

Chartered Society of Physiotherapy, www.csp.org.uk, 020 7306 6666

Royal College of Psychiatrists, www.rcpsych.ac.uk, 020 7235 2351

Complementary and Natural Healthcare Council, www.cnhc.org.uk, 020 3178 2199

Contact a Family, www.cafamily.org.uk, 0808 808 3555

Down's Syndrome Medical Interest Group, www.dsmig.org.uk

Educdation and Resources for Improving Childhood Continence, www.eric.org.uk, 0845 370 8008

Food Standards Agency, www.food.gov.uk, 07823 445801

General Regulatory Council For Complementary Therapies, www.grcct.org, 0870 3144031

Health and Care Professionals Council (for the register for physiotherapists, occupational therapists, dieticians, speech and language therapists), www.hpc-uk.org, 0845 300 6184

Hope2Sleep, www.hope2sleepguide.co.uk

KLS Support UK, www.kls-support.org.uk

National Autistic Society, www.autism.org.uk, 0808 8004104

National Institute for Health and Clinical Excellence (NICE), www.nice.org.uk, 0845 003 7780

Nursing and Midwifery Council, www.nmc-uk.org, 020 7637 7181

Royal College of Speech and Language Therapists, www.rcslt.org, 020 7378 1200

Scope, www.scope.org.uk

Tattybumpkin, www.tattybumpkin.com, 0845 680 0480

Yogabugs, www.yogabugs.com, 0121 777 7792

Experts consulted for this book

Jane Cross is a child behaviour expert at Behaviour Advice: www.behaviouradvice.co.uk.

Dr Kairen Cullen is an educational psychologist who has worked with many children and their families to offer guidance around learning. Dr Cullen is frequently featured in the national media as an expert in her field and we thank her for offering her time to our research. More details about Dr Cullen may be found at www.drkairencullen.com.

Clare Earley is a sleep practitioner for The Children's Sleep Charity as well as a mum of a child with additional needs who once had sleep issues.

Dr Heather Elphick is a paediatrician at Sheffield Children's Hospital. She runs the sleep clinic at the hospital which offers a full range of sleep monitoring and treatments. www.sheffieldchildrens.nhs.uk

Helen Gill is a specialist speech and language therapist and owns Time4talking, a company specializing in supporting the development of communication for children with additional needs. www.time4talking.co.uk

Kath Hope is the founder of Hope2Sleep and a sufferer of sleep apnoea. Her website contains information about sleep apnoea: www.hope2sleep.co.uk. There is also a friendly forum at www.hope2sleepguide.co.uk and a sleep apnoea blog at www.sleepapnoeablog.com.

Emma Sweet is a sleep practitioner specializing in behavioural interventions. Emma is a sleep expert on Channel 4's Bedtime Live series and a volunteer for The Children's Sleep Charity. She is also an occupational therapist and runs a sleep service in Northamptonshire.

Eileen Jacques is the information and helpline manager from ERIC, the only national children's charity dedicated to supporting children, young people and their families with wetting and soiling problems. www.eric.org.uk

Sue King is a paediatric physiotherapist for Kingkraft. www.kingkraft.co.uk

Dr Louise Langman is a clinical psychologist with an expertise in family therapy. Dr Langman also specializes in autism spectrum disorders and offers support directly to parents as well as undertaking medico-legal work. More details about Dr Langman can be found at www.achippp.org.uk/directory/psychologist/228.

Dr Andrew Mayers is a senior lecturer in clinical psychology and statistics at Bournemouth University. He has a specialist interest in sleep and runs sleep workshops in local schools. www.andrewmayers.info

Sarah Newbury MRPharmS is a pharmacist.

Composer Catherine Rannus from Belightful Music has produced two tracks for the Children's Sleep Charity. She continues to research how frequencies within music can impact on mood. www.belightfulmusic.co.uk

Julie Sutton is an independent disability nurse and sleep practitioner training for the Handsel Project.

Marneta Viegas is director of Relax Kids and a leading expert in child-relaxation techniques. Relax Kids have developed a range of relaxation products including books and CDs. www.relaxkids.com

Lynn Wilshaw is a Relate licensed counsellor. www.lynnwilshaw.co.uk

Reading List

Sleep Difficulties and Autism Spectrum Disorders: A Guide for Parents and Professionals, Kenneth J. Aitken (JKP, 2012)

Sleep Better: A Guide to Improving Sleep for Children with Special Needs, V. Mark Durand (Brookes, 1997)

Special Educational Needs: A Parent's Guide, Antonia Chitty and Victoria Dawson (Need2Know, 2008)

Down's Syndrome: The Essential Guide, Antonia Chitty and Victoria
Dawson (Need2Know, 2010)
Food and Your Special Needs Child, Antonia Chitty and Victoria
Dawson (Robert Hale, 2013)
Solving Children's Sleep Problems: A Step by Step Guide for Parents,
Lyn Quine (Beckett Karlson, 1997)
*The Journey Through Assessment: Help for Parents with a Special
Needs Child*, Antonia Chitty and Victoria Dawson (Robert Hale,
2013)

Endnotes

1 Bartlett, L.B., Rooney, V. and Spedding, S. (1985), 'Nocturnal difficulties in a population of mentally handicapped children', *British Journal of Mental Subnormality*; 31: 54–9. Cited in McDaid C. and Sloper P., (2008), 'Evidence on Effectiveness of Behavioural Interventions to Help Parents Manage Sleep Problems in Young Disabled Children': University of York; Social Policy Research Review; C4EO; p. 1.

2 Richdale, A.L. and Prior, M.R. (1995), 'The sleep/wake rhythm in children with autism', *European Child and Adolescent Psychiatry*; 4: 175–286.

3 Polimeni, M.A., Richdale, A.L. and Francis, A.J.P. (2005), 'A survey of sleep problems in autism, Asperger's disorder and typically developing children', *Journal of Intellectual Disability Research*, 49: 260–68. DOI: 10.1111/j.1365-2788.2005.00642.x.

4 Wiggs, L. and Stores, G. (1996), 'Sleep problems in children with severe intellectual disabilities: what help is being provided?', *Journal of Applied Research in Intellectual Disabilities*; 9:159–64.

5 Brotherton, A.M., Abbott, J., and Aggett, P.J. (2007), 'The impact of percutaneous endoscopic gastrostomy feeding in children: the parental perspective', *Child: Care, Health and Development*, 33:539–46.

6 Hallbook, T., Lundgren, J. and Rosén, I. (2007), 'Ketogenic diet improves sleep quality in children with therapy-resistant epilepsy' *Epilepsia*, Vol: 48, Issue: 1, pp. 59–65.

7 Blunden, S.L., Milte, C.M. and Sinn N. (2011), 'Diet and sleep in children with attention deficit hyperactivity disorder: preliminary data in Australian children', *J. Child Health Care*, Mar;15(1):14–24.

8 Pelsser, L.M., Frankena, K., Buitelaar, J.K. and Rommelse, N.N. (2010), 'Effects of food on physical and sleep complaints in children with ADHD: a randomised controlled pilot study', *European*

Journal of Pediatrics, Sep;169(9):1129-38. DOI: 10.1007/s00431-010-1196-5. Epub: 17 April 2010.

9 Kemp, A. (2008), 'Food additives and hyperactivity', *British Medical Journal,* May 24; 336(7654): 1144.

10 Palmer S., Rapoport J. and Quinn S. (1975), 'Food additives and hyperactivity', *Clinical Pediatrics,* 14; (10):956–9.

11 www.nhs.uk/conditions/food-additive-intolerance/Pages/Introduction.aspx, accessed 12.03.2013.

12 Galland, B.C. and Mitchell, E.A. (2010), 'Review: helping children sleep', *Archives of Disease in Childhood,* 95:850–53, DOI:10.1136/adc.2009.162974.

13 Dworak, M., Wiaterb, A., Alferc, D., Stephanc, E., Hollmannd, W., Strüder, H.K. (2008), 'Increased slow-wave sleep and reduced Stage 2 sleep in children depending on exercise intensity', *Sleep Medicine,* Volume 9, Issue 3, March, pp. 266–72.

14 Dworak, M., Schierl, T., Bruns, T. and Strüder, H.K. (2007), 'Impact of Singular Excessive Computer Game and Television Exposure on Sleep Patterns and Memory Performance of School-aged Children', *Pediatrics,* Vol. 120, No. 5, November 1, pp. 978–85, DOI: 10.1542/peds.2007-0476.

15 Babineau, S. and Goodwin, C. (2008), 'Medications for Insomnia Treatment in Children', *American Family Physician,* Feb 1;77(3):358–9.

16 MHRA/CHM Advice – March 2008, Feb 2009.

17 Babineau, S. and Goodwin, C. (2008), 'Medications for Insomnia Treatment in Children', *American Family Physician,* Feb 1;77(3):358–9.

18 Furman, C.E. (1978), 'The effect of musical stimuli on the brain-wave production of children', *Journal of Music Therapy,* Vol. 15, pp. 108–17.

19 Jackson, J.T. and Owens, J.L. (1999), 'A stress management classroom tool for teachers of children with BD', *Intervention in School and Clinic,* 35(2), 74–8.

20 Lewith, G.T., Godfrey, A.D. and Prescott, P. (2005), *The Journal of Alternative and Complementary Medicine,* August, 11(4): 631–7, DOI:10.1089/acm.2005.11.631.

21 Williams, T.I. (2006), 'Evaluating Effects of Aromatherapy

Massage on Sleep in Children with Autism: A Pilot Study', *Evidence-Based Complementary and Alternative Medicine,* vol. 3, no. 3, pp. 373–7, DOI:10.1093/ecam/nel017.

22 Shur-Fen Gau, S. (2006), 'Prevalence of sleep problems and their association with inattention/hyperactivity among children aged 6–15 in Taiwan', *Journal of Sleep Research,* Dec;15(4):403-14.

Index